About the authors

Emma Haslett and Gabriella Griffith met while working as business journalists, and bonded over their fondness for bright lipstick and their loathing for confusing corporate doublespeak. They launched their podcast, Big Fat Negative, in August 2018, in an effort to wrangle the equally confusing doublespeak surrounding infertility and IVF, and debunk some myths while they were at it. The podcast, which mixes a humorous take on infertility with expert interviews, has received wide acclaim, with mentions on BBC *Woman's Hour*, the *Telegraph*, the *Metro*, and Refinery 29.

BIG
FAT
NEGATIVE

Emma Haslett & Gabriella Griffith

PIATKUS

PIATKUS

First published in Great Britain in 2022 by Piatkus

9 10 8

Copyright © Emma Haslett and Gabriella Griffith 2022

The moral right of the author has been asserted.

A CIP catalogue record for this book
is available from the British Library.

ISBN 978-0-349-42732-4

Typeset in Sabon by M Rules
Printed and bound in Great Britain by Clays Ltd, Elcograf S.p.A

Papers used by Piatkus are from well-managed forests
and other responsible sources.

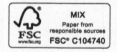

Piatkus
An imprint of
Little, Brown Book Group
Carmelite House
50 Victoria Embankment
London EC4Y 0DZ

An Hachette UK Company
www.hachette.co.uk

www.littlebrown.co.uk

To Noah and Otis, who were worth the wait,
and to Mr Emma and Mr Gabby, whose
great ideas we don't listen to enough.

Contents

Introduction:
'Tell Us About Your *Jourrrney*'

Since 2018 we've put on our best *Valley Girl* vocal fry to kick off almost 100 episodes of our podcast, Big Fat Negative, with the phrase 'Tell us about your *jourrrney*'– and everyone's told us something different.

Perhaps our interviewee is there after years of trying for a baby naturally but hasn't quite decided whether the next step – IVF, adoption, surrogacy or something else – is right for them. Perhaps they've arrived on our show after multiple pregnancy losses drove them to speak out. Maybe they were diagnosed with something at a young age and realised that they needed to start thinking about a baby at a stage in life when most of their friends' main worries are about hangover remedies. Perhaps they're in a same-sex couple and they have been plunged straight into the confusing world of sperm donors and ovulation induction.

What stands out are the common experiences. We've heard dozens of stories about the friends who shrug and say, 'I think maybe you'd find it easier if you just *relaxed* a bit?', or the cousins who swear their best friend spent years trying, then finally got pregnant when she went on holiday, or the colleagues who barge into a whispered, private conversation to recommend acupuncture ('my wife swore by it'), or the friends' husbands who lurch over at a barbecue specifically to quip, 'I heard you're trying for a baby. Do you want my kids? They're yours if you want them, ha ha.' Those with a faith have been told, 'It's God's will'; those without have been told, 'It's fate'; those who have lost babies have been told, 'It just wasn't meant to be' or 'At least you know you can get pregnant.'

Then there's the gut-punch that happens when yet another friend breezily announces their pregnancy. If you've struggled to conceive, you'll know how it feels to be doing your best to be happy for this person you love and their life-changing news, but knowing, deep down, that you're about to lose another ally to the Mum Club. The creeping knowledge that when your longed-for child *does* eventually come, it'll be so much younger than your friends' kids – those imagined days watching your children play together are vanishing as those kids grow.

Finally, there's the confusion: the alphabet soup of Internet forums, full of talk about OPKs and FMU and AF and TTC. WTF are they on about? Why are they so insistent about pineapple? What exactly is sperm-friendly lube? And how is it possible that a place designed to support one another is so bloody *cliquey*? (Don't worry, we'll be explaining all those abbreviations.)

We started the Big Fat Negative (BFN) podcast because we needed a space to vent; a place where no one was going to tell us to relax or try to solve our problems. We were both pretty sure that our problems were beyond home remedies (no amount of gong baths or yoga sessions were going to solve blocked Fallopian tubes or male-factor infertility brought on by an adolescent bout of mumps). We needed a place to *laugh*, too. It's frustrating when your friends are trying to be so kind and empathetic: they can't laugh at your story about wearing a jumpsuit to an internal examination, or racing through the streets of London with a vial of sperm.

With backgrounds in journalism, we also wanted to find a way to cut through the crap you read on the Internet and find out from experts what was actually true and what was just old wives' tales. Fertility has so much mysticism around it, but what does the science say? A podcast seemed like a very good excuse to find out. We've interviewed hormone specialists, embryologists, gynaecologists, acupuncturists, urologists, grief counsellors – you name it – all in a mission to understand infertility, IVF and the trials of trying for a baby.

This book is an extension of our podcast: it's designed to make you feel less alone by telling you our stories, telling you other people's stories and giving you solid facts about what will (and what definitely won't) help you bring home your baby. In some chapters you'll find us myth busting (explaining which myths are true and which are false), in others, we'll be seeking practical advice and reassurance from the experts. (Spoiler alert: we're not experts.)

You'll find chapters explaining the practical side of trying to conceive (TTC), from how your menstrual cycle works, how to track ovulation and preparing your body for pregnancy to getting a diagnosis, male-factor infertility, organising and going through fertility treatment and how to navigate a pregnancy loss. We'll also look at how infertility affects your life, with chapters on working while trying for a baby, how to maintain your friendships and what our partners can do to help.

The book is more than the sum of its parts: it's also about

destroying the taboo. We want to help you understand that although it might not feel like it, you're going through the same thing as millions of people out there. One in six couples has trouble conceiving, and that figure doesn't even take into account the single people who go through fertility treatment. This means that millions of people are probably feeling the same way as you right now. They're just not, for whatever reason, talking about it.

That's our call to action: read this book, hear our stories, then if you feel you can, go out and share yours. You don't have to tell the world. Find the friend or relative who is feeling the same pain as you, because we can guarantee to you that you have one, and start a conversation with them. Find your space to vent.

Take it from two idiots who started a podcast because they needed a reason to talk about it: things get easier when you tell us about your *jourrrney*.

Good luck out there.

Gabby and Emma x

A note on language We know that the way people experience infertility, and the people who experience infertility, is as varied as humanity itself. We have tried to tell as many stories as possible in this book, although we haven't managed to include everyone's experience – not by a long shot. Similarly, we know that not all women own a uterus, and not everyone who owns a uterus identifies as a 'woman', but in this book we tend to use the word 'women' as a shorthand for those who do own uteruses, and who, by virtue of that fact, undergo the most prodding, poking and treatment when it comes to fertility. We have also included a chapter about 'men', which obviously is applicable to anyone who does, or who hopes to, produce sperm. We hope that most of the advice can be applied, where relevant, to all those who need it.

Another note on language The world of infertility is jam-packed with confusing acronyms and medical terminology. Whether you're scouring TTC forums, talking to your doctors about your upcoming procedures (HyCoSy, anyone?) or trying to find a way to say how far into your TWW (two-week wait) you are (2dp5dt, yeah?) – it can make your head spin. To help, we've compiled a handy glossary. You can find this at the back starting on page 295, but feel free to flick ahead to it as you read.

Meet Emma

When I was eight years old, my brother was born. My sister, who was three years younger than me, had been fine as a sibling, because she had quickly become a sort of minion who could be trained to perform acts of vandalism and/or terrorism, and then made to take the blame when it was discovered. This new one, though – all he did was cry and vomit. When one of my mum's friends showed up at our house with a present for him and not for me, I made a decision: I *hated* babies.

All through my teens and into my twenties, while my friends were cooing over some kid, I was pulling faces. Babies were boring and gross. They didn't shake hands, which was frankly rude, and they had absolutely no chat. I'd much rather spend my life building my career and going on holiday and buying beautiful things, and maybe having a small dog, if it came to that, than ruining everything over one of these mewling, shitting, whining creatures.

Then one day, when I was in my mid-twenties, a friend of mine became the latest to announce her pregnancy. It was pretty standard for that period: everyone and their mum was getting knocked-up. But this time, the creeping sensation of envy I had begun to experience during these announcements overwhelmed me. I went home and cried. I couldn't figure out *why*; could it be that, actually, I might want a baby?

A couple of years later, shortly after we got married, Mr Emma's cousin sent us an email about Robertsonian translocation, the chromosomal disorder Mr Emma was a carrier of, which increases the likelihood of pregnancy loss or conceiving a child with a disorder such as Down's syndrome. She laid out the facts and what she had been through to conceive her son. We knew he had it. What we hadn't realised was quite how hard it could make it for us to fall pregnant.

She recommended an appointment with a genetics counsellor so that we could assess our options. Suddenly, that vague notion that I might want a baby became a blaring alarm: I needed something in my arms. We had planned to start trying a year after we got married, but suddenly I was absolutely sure that I wanted a baby – and I wanted it *now*.

What happened next is, I imagine, deeply relatable: while we awaited an appointment with the genetics counsellor – and then a referral for IVF – we decided to try naturally. That went very quickly from 'a full and healthy sex life' to obsessive googling, precision-timed sex and an addiction to peeing on sticks as I became increasingly frustrated that nothing was happening. This wasn't supposed to happen: the translocation was supposed to increase the chances of pregnancy loss and having a baby with chromosomal problems. It wasn't supposed to prevent me from getting pregnant altogether.

In my desperation to avoid IVF, I tried everything: apps, ovulation kits, measuring my body temperature every morning and putting it on a chart ('perhaps if I put it on physical graph paper rather than an app it'll be me manifesting it more?'), sperm-friendly lube, gallons of raspberry leaf tea and tons of pineapple. My period had taken ages to come back after I had gone off the Pill, and when it did come back, it was very irregular, so I found a (pretty dodgy) doctor who prescribed me three rounds of Clomid in an effort to force ovulation, no questions asked.

It was only after my GP took pity on me and began proper investigations that I discovered the appendicitis I had had when I was 11, which led to an infection of the lining of my abdomen called peritonitis, had scarred my Fallopian tubes so badly that they didn't function. They were impassable, like a mountain road in the winter.

What followed was years of treatment and the learning of many acronyms and jargon terms: two uncomfortable HSGs, a procedure in which a doctor attempts to flush dye through the Fallopian tubes to see if they are open; two laparoscopies (keyhole surgeries to assess the condition of my Fallopian tubes), which resulted in their removal; innumerable scans and blood tests; one egg collection; a failed embryo transfer; three cancelled cycles; and one transfer – which led to a successful pregnancy. From going off the Pill to the birth of my daughter, it was about four years.

Along the way, I complained *bitterly* to anyone who would listen (and to a lot of people who wouldn't). A lot of people told me to 'just relax', quite a few offered me their kids (it got a bit awks after I said, 'Cool – do you need me to sign something, or ... ?'). What I didn't get was much empathy. No one I knew was going through this, and those who did, didn't really understand it. I started to feel very, very alone.

Then one day, a few months after her wedding, my cool friend Gabby said that she and her husband had started trying for a baby and that it wasn't happening. I seized on the chance to say bonding things like, 'Has anyone told you to just relax yet?' '*Yes!*' she said. 'All the fucking time!'

I'd been blogging a bit about my experiences, but I had an idea for a podcast that would give me an excuse to talk to other people about theirs – and, more importantly, debunk those wild myths doing the rounds on online forums. I wanted to talk to a doctor who could tell me *why* eating pineapple would (or wouldn't) work, and where the rumour came from; I wanted someone medical to tell me what exactly constituted the first day of my period. And I wanted to do it all in the company of someone who could see the funny side of this ridiculous situation: I needed a co-host who was good at jizz jokes.

As luck would have it, not only had Gabby's husband given her a podcast mic for Christmas that year, but also her ability to shoehorn gags about bodily fluids into situations that only vaguely warranted them was second to none. When we started recording in August 2018, we were staggered by the response: here was a group of women who, like me, had been going through this alone. We could be the empathetic girlfriends they didn't have. The rest, as they say, is history.

Meet Gabby

We were in a bar in Berlin when my future husband told me about the time he had the mumps and his testicle swelled to the size of a lemon. We laughed when he recalled the painful pendulum between his legs – swinging perilously every time he moved. The consequences didn't really occur to us.

Fast forward – past moving in together, getting a couple of cats, throwing some banging parties in our Peckham bungalow, going on some amazing holidays – we eventually decided to get married and, given that loads of our friends had babies by now, we decided to try for one, too.

I wasn't completely in the dark about infertility. Luckily for me, my great friend Emma was already balls-deep in her first round of IVF (such a trendsetter), so I had heard her talk about the procedures she was going through and had noted her avoiding the punch at my parties.

Naturally, when six months had passed with no double line, I moaned to her about it. When a year had passed without a BFP (big fat positive), I worked up the courage to say: 'Hey, if you ever do that infertility podcast you've mentioned making, maybe

I could be a guest?' Thankfully, she said, 'Why don't you host it with me, mate?'

With 12 months of no baby action under our belt, I felt that Mr Gabby and I could officially say we were struggling to conceive. That lemon anecdote from our first holiday together became a lot more important all of a sudden. We went to the GP to have the initial tests. I came back fairly normal – Mr Gabby, less so. After a quick look at his results, a lovely lady at Fertility Network UK, said unceremoniously, 'You'll have to have IVF.'

At the time this felt devastating. But I've since come to realise that having an identifiable problem is quite handy: we were referred to a clinic straight away rather than being told to go away and keep trying. We entered the somewhat confusing world of male-factor infertility.

On one hand, we were offered a round of IVF immediately. On the other, we were told we could *probably* still conceive naturally, so while we prepared ourselves for the potential of needles and hormones, we also kept going with apps, ovulation tests, sperm-friendly lube and a whole lot of unspontaneous shagging.

With the knowledge I had from the podcast, I was keen for my hubby to see a urologist and understand if there was anything we could do to improve his sperm health (even if that would just give us a better chance at a successful round of IVF). We paid for private urology consultations and sent Mr Gabby off to have further tests. All our explorations came back normal so we kept going for a bit longer. 'You never know! Maybe we'll be one of those couples who get pregnant just before they start their injections!'

Reader: we weren't. I got my period on Christmas Day of 2018 and started injections the next day. We would do ICSI IVF (aka intra-cytoplasmic sperm injection), where they eyeball the best-looking sperm and inject it directly into the egg, rather than sticking them all together in a Petri dish (which is what happens with regular IVF). From 21 eggs, 11 fertilised with Mr Gabby's swimmers and we ended up with five blastocyst embryos.

I was at risk of something called ovarian hyperstimulation syndrome (OHSS) and so they were reluctant to put an embryo straight back in. OHSS can make you very ill, and the presence of pregnancy hormones makes it way worse, so our five little guys went into the deep freeze. We waited a couple of cycles, and on 1 April we defrosted one and popped it back in. Eleven days later we saw our very first positive pregnancy test. Our son, Otis, was born in December 2019.

Turning our struggles to conceive into a podcast was one of the best decisions we ever made. On a terribly selfish level, when I was in the throes of it, having an outlet for my frustrations, sadness and endless dildocam jokes, was a godsend. But more than that, creating Big Fat Negative has helped people all over the world who are also struggling to conceive to feel less alone. Well, you know what they say – when life gives you lemons . . .

Meet Professor Tim

When we started the podcast, one of our most important aims was to find someone who could bust all the myths we heard on forums about getting pregnant.

Step forward, Professor Tim Child, a consultant gynaecologist and subspecialist in reproductive medicine and surgery at the Oxford University Hospitals NHS trust and the medical director at Oxford Fertility, who has been working in IVF since 1996.

Since the first episode of the podcast, Professor Tim has gamely answered our questions on everything from stress to acupuncture and supplements to whether eating McDonald's chips after embryo transfer is going to do anything to help it stick (to paraphrase Tim: 'obviously not'). For almost 100 episodes he's been generous with his time, he's taken even our maddest questions seriously – and with his soothing baritone, he's become something of a heartthrob to our podcast listeners in the process.

He has also kindly agreed to help us with this book, continuing to bust myths and making sure that we've got the science right.

When he isn't helping people to bring their baby home, Professor Tim spends his days playing guitar and singing in a band called Mo' Mojo, and racing his Caterham. His favourite colour is blue (we know because we asked).

1

Are You Sure You're Doing it Right?

(Emma)

You've decided to have a baby – may I be the first to say congratulations. And also commiserations: if you've bought this book, I'm guessing that it isn't going as smoothly as you hoped it would. I can't imagine that telling you that over 80 per cent of couples will conceive within a year, while another half of the remainder will conceive during the second year of trying, will help much either.

I tell anyone who will listen that for me the first year or two of trying to conceive were the hardest. The uncertainty, the cycle of hope and grief and hope again, and the unhelpful comments from all and sundry (quite a lot more on which later) – not to mention the weird, mechanical sex – all combined to make it a horrible, frustrating period of time (and also time for periods).

In this chapter I'll guide you through the basics of infertility, from what you need to know about your body and conception, while Gabby and sex therapist Shirlee Kay will join us briefly to talk sex while trying to conceive, and hopefully offer some reassurance about your increasingly unromantic bedtime antics. Don't panic: we're here to help.

What you'll find in this chapter:

- The hope zone, and why the emotional rollercoaster is normal.
- A quick note on 'just relax'.
- Keeping the love alive.
- The basics of TTC.
- No, really – are you sure you're doing it right?
- How to track your cycles.
- Spotting and what it means.
- Myth busting: legs in the air.

My story

I like to think of myself as a realist. When I first started TTC, I had an inkling that there might be a problem: something to do with the multiple little slip-ups that had not yielded the dire consequences my sex ed. teacher had warned me about. That, plus the email from Mr Emma's cousin indicating that the chromosomal disorder he is a carrier of wasn't quite as unimportant as we had thought.

Nevertheless, having spent our honeymoon planning married life ('We'll spend the first year just having a lovely time together, then we'll get pregnant the following January and then we'll do it again about 18 months later – two years is *such* a lovely age gap, don't you think?'), I dutifully ditched the Pill around our first wedding anniversary, then waited for my period to arrive. And waited. And waited – for six months.

While I waited, I began to obsessively scrutinise my body. Perhaps my period hadn't come because I was pregnant? Was it my imagination or were my boobs sorer than usual? Was that a metallic taste in my mouth? I took pregnancy test after pregnancy test. Quite often I dug them out of the bin the next day, just to check that a second line hadn't mysteriously developed overnight.

When my period did finally show up, I thought: *This is it – I'm definitely going to get pregnant now.* I started ovulation testing because that's what people on the Internet did, and also my cousin had said that it worked for her friend. A couple of months later when I still wasn't pregnant I started taking my temperature every morning and putting the result into an app, because someone had said *that* magically got you knocked up, and I was beginning to get a bit frustrated.

After months of becoming increasingly obsessed with my cycle, I had a tearful appointment with my GP, who agreed something probably wasn't right and referred me for fertility testing. But not before one of my 'hilarious' friends joked: 'Are you sure you're doing it right?'

The hope zone

One of the things people who become pregnant at the drop of a hat don't often understand is what an emotional roller-coaster it can be. While she was in the early stages of fertility treatment, Gabby came up with the concept of emotional 'zones' during TTC, and I kicked myself, because I wished I'd thought of it first. It goes like this: you start in the 'hope zone', the period of optimism during the couple of weeks after ovulation, which is usually spent mooching past the doorways of baby shops and idly thinking of names that are 'unusual but not weird', like Hugo and Ophelia. Next comes the 'disappointed zone': this is either delivered on the incoming tide of your period, or a little earlier if you've taken a pregnancy test. The hope drains from you like sand in an egg timer. Depending on how long you've been trying, you could feel a touch of disappointment and a bit silly for having dared to believe, but then you carry on, or you spend a week sobbing, giving pregnant women the evil eye and stuffing your face with ice cream.

Finally, comes the 'determined zone', where you gather your thoughts, assess when your next fertile window will be, and in many cases spend quite a lot of money on Amazon on things like sperm-friendly lube and ovulation kits, just to make super-sure that you're ready next time.

Everyone reading this book will have experienced a month (or cycle) where they are *convinced* that they are pregnant. All the evidence points that way: sore boobs, odd dreams – and do your nipples look a *teeny* bit darker? Is your uterus feeling a bit . . . stretchy?

Then you take a pregnancy test and – lo! There's only one line. Of *course* there's only one line. But could the pregnancy test be wrong? Just to make you feel a bit better, here's a list of things I did to be *extra sure* that another line wasn't actually there and I just couldn't see it:

- Looked at the test in four different rooms, to make sure that the line I thought I saw definitely *was* just a shadow.
- Took a photo of the test and zoomed in.

- Took a photo of the test and added a polarising filter, because the Internet said sometimes you can see faint lines better that way.
- Dug the test out of the bin the next morning, to make sure a second line hadn't appeared overnight (it happened to someone on the Internet).
- Dug the test out of the bin the next morning, then pulled the test apart, to make sure the second line wasn't hiding inside the casing (it happened to someone on the Internet) (this behaviour is also known as rock bottom).

What I'm trying to say is that ups and downs and strange behaviours are completely normal. Don't waste energy beating yourself up for feeling this way. You are not mad.

'Just relax'

Many years ago, a scientist somewhere decided that it was a great idea to study the effect of stress on conception. What followed was decades and decades of people who have never had trouble popping out sprogs telling their infertile friends increasingly creative variations on 'just relax and it will happen'.

One of my low points came when I was fairly early on in the process of trying to conceive. Following yet another evening of 'reassuring' stories about a friend's cousin's dog's sister's owner's mate who had been trying for 'like, *decades*' but then got magically knocked up while on holiday, I turned to my only TTC friend: an Internet forum. 'Does anyone else keep being told to relax?' I asked. 'Is it the most annoying thing in the world?' The answers weren't encouraging: 'It worked for me,' shrugged one respondent. Right, OK.

The fact is, no one has ever relaxed when they've been told to relax. And actually, 'just relax' is a form of victim blaming: it's implying your inability to conceive is your fault. We'll cover stress and people's responses in the next chapter, but for now I want you to understand that *being stressed about the situation is very unlikely to be preventing you from getting pregnant*. Banish that idea from your head immediately.

There now. Don't you feel more relaxed already?

Gabby on keeping the love alive

Ah, procreation: the miracle of life. It's the reason we're all here, after all: that primal, visceral urge to make a baby. If you're in a heterosexual relationship, after a while, procreation also has a tendency to become the biggest mood killer known to man (and woman).

I remember this time with Technicolor vividness. When I first started trying for a baby, the sex was great. It had this whole new layer of meaning that it hadn't had before. I'd lie there afterwards smiling to myself – 'Was that the one?' I would book nice hotels to go away for a baby-making retreat and think about increasingly ridiculous baby names relating to the hotel or place (Conrad and Osaka were real contenders after a trip to Japan). It was an exciting time.

But it didn't last. Soon I was reaching for the fertility tracker apps – logging shags instead of cuddling after sex. I quickly realised that you don't have sex when you feel sexy, you have sex when a little notification from your app pops up on your phone, or when an ovulation stick smiles at you. Nudge nudge, wink wink – get shagging! Is there any greater mood killer than telling your partner you have to 'Do *it* NOW – *the app says DO IT NOW!*'?

Eventually, I remember looking at my husband and simply seeing a walking sperm. He had what I needed. I just needed to top up on sperm and then I'd be good for that day. Ovulation, tick. Spermy top-ups, tick. Pregnancy assured. Except – spoiler alert – it wasn't.

The problem is that sex 'becomes almost mechanical', says Shirlee Kay, a therapist who specialises in couples, sex and fertility. 'It does change the dynamics of how couples are having sex.' She says that couples might have to accept that for the time being things won't be as magical as they once were. 'Surrender to that space. Don't create this idea that it has to be romantic. When you let go of that, some of the spontaneity, some of the ability to just have fun in that space is possible.'

Guilt is a real problem around the entire TTC process, but dragging partners into sex doesn't make things any easier. 'Women feel very guilty about it,' says Shirlee, but it takes two to tango. 'Actually, it's a joint thing, so you have to really get on the same page and have that conversation that "this is for both of us".' Couples should accept that 'it is going to kill our sex life for the time being, but let's do what we have to do to get pregnant, and then kind of reconnect'.

Whatever you do, don't do extra work by trying to 'keep things flirty'. All those articles suggesting that you 'send sexy texts' to your partner on ovulation day, or have sex outside your fertile window 'for fun'? Do it if you feel like it, but not if it feels like a chore. 'It's contrived,' says Shirlee. 'It is not being authentic. Intimacy is about being real, it's about being in your body, knowing that you're going through fertility treatment or just trying to conceive, and that your body's kind of tense. Work with that information.'

TTC: the very, very basics

Right, it's Emma, I'm back. Now we've talked about what's going on in your head, let's look at what's happening in your body. You at the back, sit up straight, because I'm about to explain how a woman's menstrual cycle works. Or how it's *supposed* to work.

The first day of your period is the first day of your cycle. Over the next few days, the uterus sheds the lining it has lovingly built up.

Once the period has finished, a few follicles (fluid-filled sacs) in the ovaries, each containing an egg, start to mature and grow in size. A few days later, the follicle with the biggest, juiciest egg (the 'leading' follicle) pops and the egg moves into the Fallopian tube then waits for between 12 and 24 hours for a sperm to rock up. This is called ovulation.

If a sperm appears, it burrows into the egg and they become an embryo. After a few days, that makes its way through the rest of the Fallopian tube, plops into the uterus, finds a lovely soft bit of lining to attach itself to and makes itself comfortable for the next nine months or so.

It's also worth discussing what hormones are doing during all this, because hormone levels are how both home-test kits and blood tests determine whether everything is working properly.

There are four hormones playing different roles during the menstrual cycle. Follicle stimulating hormone (FSH), produced by the pituitary gland, does what it says on the tin: kicking things off by causing an egg to develop in the follicle. The maturing ovarian follicle releases oestrogen, which causes the uterine lining to thicken. It peaks just before the egg is released, when lutenising hormone (LH), also produced in the pituitary gland, jumps, triggering the release of the egg.

Once the egg is released, the empty follicle becomes what is known as a corpus luteum, releasing progesterone, which helps the uterine lining to thicken further. If the egg is fertilised and attaches itself to the lining (that is, you get pregnant) it will release human chorionic gonadotropin (hCG), the hormone pregnancy tests look for, and progesterone levels will continue to climb for the first 12 weeks of pregnancy (after which the placenta will take over). If not, progesterone falls right down around day 28, and the cycle begins again.

It's worth pointing out that most pregnancy tests can detect an hCG level of over 10mIU/ml (that's milli-international units per millilitre). At that point, you'll get a faint positive, which will (hopefully) darken over the following days as the amount of hCG released by the growing embryo increases. In a healthy pregnancy the amount of hCG being produced by the embryo should double every 48 hours or so.

Occasionally the embryo will stop growing very early on and the amount of hCG will fall, which is why the Internet is so obsessed with how dark pregnancy test lines are. If that happens, it is rather dismissively called a chemical pregnancy. If you haven't tested, you will think your period is a little late. If you have tested and you're anything like us, you'll be devastated, but everyone will try to comfort you with unhelpful phrases like 'It just wasn't meant to be' and 'At least you know you can get pregnant', which will make you feel even worse.

Anyway, I digress.

No, really – are you sure you're doing it right?

In the UK, GPs are the gatekeepers to the world of fertility testing: they should be the first person you speak to when you realise that you are struggling to conceive. The first thing they will do is consult guidelines from the National Institute for Health and Care Excellence (NICE), which makes recommendations to the NHS about how to treat patients. We'll be name-checking it a lot in this book.

NICE guidelines state that 'vaginal sexual intercourse every two to three days optimises the chance of pregnancy' (not, as one of our guests' patients had it, 'four to six times a day'. Yeesh!). That's mainly to do with sperm quality: do it too infrequently and most of the sperm will be dead. Do it too frequently, and your man won't have enough time to, ahem, prepare his best men for battle.

Now, all that sounds fair enough in theory, but, practically speaking, it is quite difficult. By the time you have bought this book, you will probably have been trying to conceive for at least six months. Have you been having sex every two or three days during that period? You OK, hun? Are things becoming a little ... 'chafey' down there?

Kate Davies is a fertility nurse consultant whose private practice Your Fertility Journey helps people to understand why they aren't conceiving. She says the first thing you need to get to grips with is the fertile window: the few days during the month when you are most likely to conceive. As we have already discovered, the egg only hangs around for a day or so, so it's vital that you get this right.

Kate is very emphatic on one point: apps on your phone aren't going to help you figure out when this window is open. 'It's not going to give you the information that you need.' Even the apps themselves are beginning to recognise that. At least one major period tracker has stopped suggesting a fertile window, because it has recognised that everyone's body is different.

'The fertile window is based on the life of the egg and the life of the sperm,' says Kate. 'The egg's life is very short: 12 hours, possibly 24. The life of the sperm is a lot longer, so five days, possibly even up to seven. Therefore, you work out your fertile window based on the life of the egg and the life of the sperm. It's around about six days on average.'

Why all the vague language? Because, as we have learned, women's cycles vary so much. But one way you can work it out, and reduce the frequency of those scheduled sex sessions, is by becoming aware of when your fertile window is open.

Tracking your cycles

I'm afraid that I am going to use the terms 'cervical mucus' and 'secretions' a lot in the next few paragraphs. We might as well just get used to it, so let's say it out loud together: cervical mucus, secretions. Cervical mucus, secretions. My apologies to your fellow passengers if you're currently using public transport.

Right. Cervical mucus is the substance secreted by your cervix as your body gears up to ovulate. Any cervical mucus is a sign that oestrogen is beginning to build up as the follicles in your ovaries prepare an egg. Your body is preparing to ovulate. It has different consistencies during your cycle, which either help or hinder sperm from reaching your uterus. As you come closer to ovulation, it becomes more 'gloopy', as Kate puts it, and it's designed by your body to help sperm make it to the egg.

At the beginning of your cycle, 'If you've got it between finger and thumb, which is a way of testing, initially it would just break, you wouldn't be able to stretch it,' says Kate. '[With] fertile secretions [i.e. just before ovulation], you literally could get some between the thumb and the finger and really stretch it.'

The Internet might be full of talk of the most fertile mucus having an 'egg white' consistency around your fertile window, but Kate cautions against looking for that. 'Not everyone has that. What's really important to get to know is what is normal for you. It might be that you don't have egg-white appearance, but you feel quite damp, the secretions feel really profuse, and that is your normal fertile secretions.'

Adding more data

Cervical mucus is one factor, but the best way to figure out when (and if) you are really ovulating is by adding another data point. Kate suggests either checking your cervix or measuring your body temperature.

Checking your cervix is relatively straightforward, if a little uncomfortable. Have a feel every morning. It goes from being low in the vagina and feeling hard, like the tip of your nose, to moving up in your vagina and feeling soft, like your earlobes, during your fertile period. Over the course of a couple of cycles you will get used to its changes and be able to tell when you are ovulating.

Another way to do it (although we should point out here that NICE guidelines aren't supportive of this, so make your own decision on whether it's really worth it) is to track your temperature. There are two ways to do this:

Basal body temperature Use a thermometer that runs to at least two decimal places, and take your temperature under your tongue each morning. This is slightly tricky because you need to do it *before you do anything*: do not sit up, talk, drink or go to the loo before you take your temperature.

Core body temperature is a more invasive, if more reliable, way of doing it. The pros: this measures the temperature at which your body maintains your organs and cells, meaning that you don't have to do it before you've done anything else, although it helps to do it around the same time each day. The cons: the best way to measure your core temperature is rectally or vaginally. We'll just leave that there ...

Either way, plot your temperature on a piece of graph paper and look out for a tell-tale jump. You're looking for a notable rise in temperature. Once (if) that happens, ovulation has occurred.

One last note on fertility awareness, and particularly temperature tracking, from Kate: 'It's important to say that what you don't want to be doing is adding to any stress. So, if a woman's doing that and it's stressing her, then that's defeating the purpose.' I was definitely a casualty of this. One day, after an incident where I very nearly wet myself because I refused to get out of bed before I had taken my temperature, Mr Emma gently pointed out that it was turning me into a crazy person. I abandoned it the next day, and stuck to ovulation testing kits (pregnancy test-like strips that you pee onto around the time of ovulation, which can predict whether you are about to ovulate based on your hormone levels) to figure out when my fertile window was.

Why am I spotting?

Ah, spotting: it can become the bane of your life. There are three reasons you might be bleeding in the middle of your cycle: pregnancy (hmph), infection and hormones. The first two can be ruled out pretty easily by a pregnancy test (sorry) and a visit to your GP. The third is a little tricky.

Spotting in the middle of your cycle is very, very common, says Professor Tim. 'It's due to the very rapid change in the oestrogen and progesterone hormones around the time of ovulation. The oestrogen is dominant in the first part of the cycle, and it's there to thicken the endometrium and get it ready. And the progesterone is there in the second half of the cycle; it's there to change the endometrium into a type that's receptive for the embryo to implant. But in that middle stage, the oestrogen and progesterone are changing really quickly, so it's quite common to get a bit of mid-cycle spotting – it's actually a sign of ovulation. It's probably actually quite a positive sign, because it shows you that things are happening.'

He says that if you're getting spotting during the luteal phase (the period of time after ovulation, but before your period), that's also nothing to worry about. 'At that time, it's just that the lining of the uterus is at its thickest and is changing to more of a glandular type of endometrium from what it was in the first half, so it's just more prone to some blood, or some endometrium, coming away.'

There's a lot of talk on the Internet of 'shortened luteal phases'. The luteal phase is the period of time between ovulation and your period. This was definitely a concern for Gabby, but Professor Tim says that's a red herring: 'It had been thought previously that a shorter luteal phase might be linked to subfertility. But again, the evidence for that is just not there. That's partly because if an embryo implants, it's still implanted before menstruation.' The only time to be concerned would be if you have 'an amazingly short luteal phase of five or six days, which you basically just don't see', he says. 'Generally, menstruation still happens after the time that an embryo would have implanted. As soon as an embryo implants, it starts to produce hCG (human chorionic gonadotropin, the pregnancy hormone), and even if levels are so low that we can't trace them, those levels can still be sufficient to keep the corpus luteum alive and to keep it producing oestrogen and progesterone, and therefore to stop the period.'

Does spotting alone prevent you from getting pregnant? 'Studies have looked at whether having spotting reduces the chances of getting pregnant naturally, and it doesn't,' he says, although it's worth being aware of how much you're bleeding. 'If someone's having full-on bleeding, that's a bit different. But the usual description would more be of some spotting, and that's not being linked to changes in the chance of natural conception.'

MYTH BUSTING: Legs in the air like you just don't care

The myth Lying with your legs up against the wall will help you to get pregnant quicker.

It's one of the oldest tricks in the TTC book, but does lying back with your legs up against the wall after you have sex like a sort of crazy post-coital lollipop make any difference when you're trying to conceive?

The bust: false In short, no, says Professor Tim. 'It will make no difference at all. And that is because the direction of the vagina is actually slightly pointed towards a woman's back, it actually tilts downwards a bit anyway. Whether her legs are straight out like she's lying flat or whether the legs are straight up in the air isn't going to make any difference to the actual angle of the vagina within the pelvis, because that's not going to move; it's not going to affect the ability of sperm to get up through the cervix.'

What you *can* do is to stay lying down for a while after sex, but again, it doesn't need to be 'hours and hours', he says. 'The ejaculation happens right up near the cervix, so the sperm are off and running anyway.'

Conclusion

What's confusing about this stage of TTC is quite how much old wives' tales reign supreme. As one person said to me fairly early on in the process, 'most women would stand naked in the middle of the road if it would guarantee them a baby'. Usually, common sense is a pretty good indicator of what works and what doesn't; take stress, for example. If it really were that much of a hindrance to getting knocked up, the human race probably wouldn't have made it much beyond the 'being attacked by an angry lion' stage.

I've given you the basics of fertility awareness here, and hopefully given you a good indicator of what should be going on inside your body when you're trying to have a baby. Whether you're still at the TTC stage or skipping straight ahead to fertility treatment, it will help you to understand what doctors are looking for and why certain treatments are being advised.

Now I've brought you up to GCSE biology level (nope, I didn't remember any of it either), let's talk about getting your body into the right place to carry a baby.

2

Getting Match Fit

(Gabby)

When you're trying (and failing) to conceive, as well as crushing disappointment each month you can probably expect to get lots of unsolicited advice about how to improve your chances. This stretches from the oh-so-friendly comments from your auntie who tells you to relax and it'll happen, to the Google search results that tell you to drink pomegranate juice every day and to stop using nail polish. But what should you *actually* do and will any of it make a difference?

In this chapter we'll explore a lot of the things that people suggest and try to explain why. Spoiler alert: we don't have all the answers. There is such little evidence in this area that it is impossible at this point to say whether most of this stuff will help. But we can give you as much information as possible so that you can go and make your own decisions.

What you'll find in this chapter:

- Advice from doctors and fertility clinics.
- What the Internet will tell you to do.

- A quick look into: exercise, stress, caffeine, acupuncture, toxins and supplements.
- A word on nutrition from Melanie Brown.
- The minefield of fertility supplements.
- Myth busting: raspberry leaf tea.

My story

It was a balmy October evening and two of my closest friends were having a joint birthday party. I was drunk. My husband and I had been trying for a baby for just over a year. I was starting to feel a bit bitter about it. When I arrived at the party I noticed someone had shared a scan photo on my husband's family WhatsApp group. 'Fecking foetuses everywhere!' I exclaimed – a bit too loudly for a posh private members' club lounge. 'Everyone in the world is fucking pregnant,' I huffed, reaching for the Sauvignon Blanc. I noticed a bit of a strange look exchanged between Jane, one of the birthday girls, and her fiancé, Dan. I was probably bringing the vibe down. I made a mental note to be more jolly and not complain about my womb again.

The party moved on to a Mexican restaurant, where we ate delicious tacos and some of us, me included, drank shots of tequila. I noticed Jane (also trying for a baby) wasn't drinking and drunkenly tried to make up for my earlier outburst, 'If you were pregnant, I wouldn't be angry, I would be over the moon for you.' She smiled awkwardly and reiterated her earlier reasoning that she was just trying to be good because she was ovulating.

I woke up the next morning feeling like an absolute arse. Yes, I had a hangover – tequila ones I always find particularly pernicious – but I also had a weird feeling of shame, maybe guilt. I was embarrassed that I had the outburst. I was a bit conscious that perhaps my friends were judging me for getting so drunk while trying for a baby. And deep down, I was starting to wonder if I should rein it in.

My ethos until that point had been that I would carry on life as normal while trying. After all, I would have to stop drinking for nine months at least when I was finally successful. My step-mother had made comments about how you should cut back on drinking while trying, but I brushed it off. People get pregnant while they're drunk every damn day. How many babies in the world wouldn't exist without alcohol?! I'd say more than half.

I went through the following week at work feeling a bit down. The remnants of a temporary tattoo from the Mexican restaurant on my arm: a constant reminder of my behaviour. I got a message from Jane. She *was* pregnant and wanted to tell me first. *Burning hot shame.* I must have made her feel so uncomfortable. God damn that white wine. I resolved to behave better. I bought *It Starts with the Egg*, by Rebecca Fett, and started reading.

I didn't get too far before I read something that stayed with me. She explained that three to four months before ovulation, an egg undergoes a major transformation and this is a critical time for egg quality. This, she explained, was the brief window in which you had the potential to improve your egg quality.

Boom! I had three months until IVF started. I had picked up this book at the right time. Perhaps my previous indiscretions could pass by without repercussion. Fett advises complete abstinence from booze when you're TTC. That said, she found that there is plenty of evidence to suggest heavy drinking impacts fertility and IVF success rates but evidence about one or two drinks a week was less consistent.

As an avid fan of wine, I decided to go down the one-or-two-glasses-a-week route. I stuck to red wine (it's practically good for you and, luckily for me, it was winter). I also stopped completely as soon as I started my IVF meds. I came to really look forward to my one or two glasses a week; the rest of the time I explored the world of alcohol-free beers and wines. There are actually some good ones. This was me starting to take some action, and it felt pretty good.

I started with booze (what's the opposite of a gateway drug? My gateway anti-drug), but soon I looked at my caffeine intake, my diet (ish) and my beauty products. You'll hear me say frequently that I have no idea if any of this helped. But I knew I was in control of something, and that helped my mental health at the very least.

What the doctors will tell you about fertility health and preparing for IVF

When you finally pluck up the courage to go and see a doctor about your seeming inability to procreate, you'll probably be expecting some lifestyle advice, along with (hopefully) some tests and the gentle advice to keep shagging regularly. If you have graduated to the IVF clinic, you'll definitely be expecting some juicy clues as to how you can increase your chances of success. After all, you'd dance naked at the crossroads drinking nettle juice backwards if it meant you'd get those two little lines.

But the reality is, in the majority of cases, the most you'll get in either scenario is a mild suggestion to take it easy on booze, quit smoking and stay away from hard drugs. Not rocket science. But anyone who has read through TTC forums, consulted Dr

Google or followed a fertility influencer on Instagram (yes, these exist) will know that there seems to be a world of advice about how you should behave, shop, eat and drink if you want sperm to meet egg and stick the hell around, so why aren't the medical professions more forthcoming?

'Coming from a scientific medical background, you give advice based on what has been proven to improve the situation – it should be no different if you're talking about something like diabetes or fertility,' says Professor Tim Child. 'Yet there's so much rubbish out there written about what people should and shouldn't do with fertility – mostly based on absolutely nothing – perhaps some journalist wrote about it and people think that there must be truth in it. Coming at it from a scientific medical background, saying "people should be eating lots of this or not eating that" based on no scientific evidence is not good medicine.'

What might you hear from your fertility doctor?

We asked Professor Tim what he often says to patients: 'There are certainly some lifestyle factors that have been proven to have an impact, and people should definitely consider changing if relevant to them. Having a BMI of over 30 has been shown to increase miscarriage rates and decrease IVF success rates. Smoking is also bad: we know that it has a negative effect on ovarian reserve and has been linked to miscarriage. These are two areas we would advise action. When it comes to drinking, my personal view is that there is no evidence to suggest people should stop drinking completely during fertility treatment. We just tell people to be sensible: a glass of wine here or there won't make a difference, in my opinion.'

Of course, for some people, hearing this seemingly solid advice is not enough. Surely there are other things you can do? There are lots of reasons why people going through infertility might want to change their lifestyle, make tweaks here and there or go mad on Amazon – control is certainly one of them. Trying and failing to conceive can leave you feeling completely at the mercy of some horribly malevolent being. You've found the partner of your dreams, like they say you should; you've been having plenty of sex, like they say you should; you've been tracking your cycles, like they say you should. But it's not working, and there's nothing you can do! By researching the optimum conditions for fertility, whether you're a woman or a man, you'll come across tips and advice. Giving something up, swapping your regular this for that, adding a new step to your routine – these are positive actions that help you to feel as though you're doing something to help your situation. You're back in control. A bit.

What the Internet will tell you about fertility health and preparing for IVF

We're going to start this section by saying that if you go deep on this, really explore every little suggestion a 'health expert' or fellow infertility warrior says will increase your chances, your brain will explode. That is the technical term. You'll be overwhelmed, feel completely hopeless and woefully unprepared for what is ahead.

We definitely recommend following any advice from your doctor – beyond that, our advice is to do your research. If there's something you've heard about that you'd like to try, and if the evidence is persuasive, then consider it. Read some articles, look for research papers and if you're active in a TTC community online, ask around. You'll get a feel for whether it's worth a go. Most importantly, only do what you feel you can do. In all likelihood, you'll find a reasonably short list of changes you feel are realistic for you to make, and stick to those. In this chapter we'll look at some of the things we did, but that doesn't make our lists better than yours. They just show what we each felt we could do at the time.

In the interests of illustrating just how expansive the wild west of fertility advice can be, however, here is a list of some of the common nuggets you will probably come across:

- Quit caffeine
- Drink pomegranate juice
- Eat the core of a pineapple during your two-week wait
- Stop using nail varnish
- Stop being stressed
- Drink raspberry leaf tea
- Do acupuncture
- Eat beetroot
- Eat only organic food
- Drop drinking alcohol
- Stop exercising
- Start exercising
- Stop wearing perfume
- Try reflexology
- Change your make-up to organic
- Get rid of harsh cleaning products
- Stop riding a bike (one for the dudes)
- Switch your shampoos/conditioners to phthalate-free ones

- Don't drink out of plastic bottles
- Don't touch receipts
- Eat nuts
- Stop eating canned goods
- Have sex in the mornings
- Use sperm-friendly lube
- Don't take ibuprofen
- Stop taking hot baths (dudes again)

We won't go through all these, but we thought we'd pick up on a few that we both have experience in.

Exercise

Ask me if I exercise and I'll tell you I'm a runner. Hopefully you'll walk away thinking I run 10k at 6am every morning before heading off for an extremely productive day at work (green juice in hand, obvs). The truth is that I probably run once a week, if I have the time. But it does make me feel good. So when it came to TTC it wasn't something I was keen to give up. After all, it's my time to think about important things such as what I would do if I won the lottery, what my last meal on earth would be and exotic baby names we'll never use (when I'm letting myself go there).*

One day after work, before I'd started IVF but certainly while I was trying naturally, I ran to Emma's house. I arrived red-faced and sweaty. She mentioned that her acupuncturist told her that it was OK that she didn't like running because it creates the stress hormone cortisol. This freaked me out. Had I just fucked our chances this month by running from Putney to Notting

(*Answers: buy a theme park, ramen, Zephyr – boy or girl.)

Hill? I started doing some research and found that most studies suggested moderate exercise when you're trying for a baby is absolutely fine, so I kept running.

When I started IVF it was a different story. When you're on ovary-stimulating drugs to create as many eggs as possible, your ovaries swell and become quite tender. Running (a) isn't much fun; and (b) it can cause something called ovary torsion – where your ovaries twist around the ligaments that hold them in place. It doesn't sound like fun. I completely stopped running during this time. I also spent an entire day paranoid that I had twisted my ovaries after going to a yoga class. I hadn't, but official advice does suggest avoiding high-impact exercise, including running, jumping and intense yoga positions while on stimulating drugs. My yoga skills don't stretch to 'intense positions' so I was actually 100 per cent safe in downward dog.

Aside from when you're on the stims during an IVF cycle (the stimulation drugs you take to encourage your ovaries to do some overtime and make significantly more egg-containing follicles), moderate exercise is not just safe it's encouraged. Professor Tim certainly thinks it's a good thing: 'There's no reason why people should avoid exercise when trying to conceive. It's better to be healthy than not. A short run isn't going to increase stress hormones – quite the opposite – if people enjoy going out for a jog it would be better to do that than not.'

He does caution against very intense exercise, especially if lack of ovulation is a problem you're experiencing. 'For some women, if they're doing extreme levels of sport – training for a marathon, for example – that can lead to very low levels of body fat and an absence of ovulation and periods. Equally, even if a woman has a normal BMI but if she's doing a lot of high-intensity exercise and in the gym every day, that can switch off ovulation – it's the body trying to protect things and make sure a woman is in an ideal health range.'

A Norwegian population health study from 2009 concluded that physical activity was only associated with an increased risk of infertility when women reported high levels of intensity in their workouts. A second study presented by Lauren A. Wise, ScD, an associate professor of epidemiology at the Boston University School of Public Health, found that moderate exercise was associated with decreased time to conceive. But non-overweight women who exercised vigorously for more than five hours a week were shown to have a 32 per cent lower chance of becoming pregnant during a cycle.

All in all I'd say non-extreme exercise is a good thing. Doing IVF? Just take it a bit easier.

Stress

(Emma's here to talk about this one, it's her favourite.)
If you've been trying for a baby for long enough to pick up this book, the chances are that at least one well-meaning friend who has suddenly developed a new expertise in fertility will have shaken their head, heaved a great sigh, and told you to 'just relax!'. 'You're just going to stress yourself out by trying so hard,' they'll have said. 'Everyone knows stress stops you from getting pregnant.' You have our permission to tell that friend that they are wrong. The suggestion that your worrying about not getting knocked up is what's preventing you from doing so is almost certainly not true.

Let's start with a 2014 study published in the catchily titled journal *Population and Development Review*, which examined birth rates during the height of the war in Iraq, between 2006 and 2011. It found that the total fertility rate stayed 'remarkably stable, with apparently no change after the onset of war'. In fact, among those aged 20–24, the fertility rate increased by about 15 per cent. In other words, living in a war zone, traditionally a pretty stressful environment, doesn't seem to affect fertility rates.

What about those tabloid headlines screeching about stress and its effects on fertility? Let's examine another one from 2014, published in the journal *Human Reproduction*, which generated headlines such as 'Stress can double the risk of infertility for women' (thank you, *Daily Mail*). The study looked at two stress markers, cortisol and alpha-amylase, an enzyme produced when adrenaline levels rise, in the saliva of 401 women trying to conceive. It concluded that the third of women with the highest alpha-amylase levels had slightly lower odds of getting knocked up compared with women in the lowest third, and that they were twice as likely not to conceive in the following year.

Where to begin with this one? Firstly, it looked at only 400 couples – in the grand scheme of things, that's not a vast number. Secondly, although the study adjusted for lifestyle factors including alcohol, caffeine and smoking, women provided only two samples of saliva, at the beginning and the end of the study. So it couldn't look at whether stress levels rose progressively as women failed to get pregnant (we're going to go out on a limb and suggest perhaps they did). Thirdly, it found no correlation between levels of cortisol – the *actual hormone produced by stress* – and the time it took for them to conceive. Meanwhile, the difference between the amount of alpha-amylase produced by those in the top third and the bottom third of the cohort is described by the NHS as 'only of borderline statistical significance', so the study is, if we're honest, pretty inconclusive.

Professor Tim explains the findings a little: he points out that if you're *really* stressed, it might stop you from ovulating for a month or two, but that doesn't cause ongoing infertility: 'Obviously, many women will say that during times of stress, exams or work deadlines, whatever it might be, it will interfere with ovulation. Of course that can happen. But in terms of it stopping ovulation month after month after month after month? No. In reality that isn't going to happen. I've never seen a patient of normal weight, who is otherwise fit and well, where a lack of ovulation is purely down to stress. That wouldn't happen.'

A 2011 meta-analysis, which took into account 14 studies of just under 3,600 women undergoing a cycle of fertility treatment, looked at whether those experiencing anxiety or stress before their cycles were less likely to achieve a pregnancy. The answer? In short: nope. 'The findings of this meta-analysis should reassure women and doctors that emotional distress caused by fertility problems or other life events co-occurring with treatment will not compromise the chance of becoming pregnant,' the authors wrote in the *BMJ*. The next time your friend tries to give you their 'advice', tell them to stick that in their pipe and smoke it.

Yes, infertility causes stress. The monthly hope–grief–hope cycle will, of course, take its toll on those cortisol levels. But what you shouldn't do is stress about being stressed, or try to turn yourself into some kind of Zen master, just because your ultra-fertile mate says that's best.

What you *should* do is start finding ways to feel less out of control, either by approaching your GP about beginning tests once you've been trying for a year, or taking some of the measures below. In our experience, sitting around worrying about worrying increases stress levels. Once you've started taking action, you'll begin to feel much calmer.

Caffeine

(Emma has joined us again here.)

I didn't drink a whole cup of coffee until I was 21. For years, I hated the stuff. But as soon as I joined the working world I knew that the only way to be taken truly seriously as the adult I was becoming was to be able to join the ranks of coffee drinkers. After several months of a regime of twice-daily mochas (the gateway coffee), I finally grew to appreciate it.

These days I love coffee. I love the smell of it, I love the taste of it, I love the ritual surrounding it. Nothing makes me happier than finding a café, ordering a latte (never skinny – people, don't ruin it) and spending half an hour savouring it while thinking about nothing in particular. The more pretentious the café, the more joy I derive from it. I can genuinely say I love having conversations about Brazilian bean varieties with moustachioed baristas.

When I booked a visit to a nutritionist as a way to get my head in the game ahead of my second frozen embryo transfer (FET), I wasn't prepared for her to tell me to cut down on the caffeine. But tell me she did, although she allowed me to stay on one cup a day because my working day began at 6.30am and she felt sorry for me. Three cancelled FETs later, though, and I had given up caffeine altogether. And do you know what? Even ditching that one cup of coffee a day gave me headaches, muscle aches and unbelievable fatigue, symptoms which all went on for well over a fortnight, which just goes to show that caffeine is just like any other mind-altering drug – we just don't tend to give it the respect it deserves.

Why all the caffeine hate from the infertility community? Ask any practitioner (acupuncturists, nutritionists, and so on) and they'll tell you that caffeine narrows your blood vessels, which in a fertility context reduces blood flow to the uterus.

Studies on the matter are conflicting. NHS guidelines recommend that pregnant women (and thus those trying to conceive) should have no more than 200mg of caffeine a day, which equates to about two cups of instant coffee. But a 2017 meta-analysis published in the journal *Clinical Epidemiology* found no 'clear' association between caffeine consumption and the chance of achieving pregnancy among couples trying to conceive, either naturally or through fertility treatment.

So far so encouraging for me and my barista friends. Unfortunately, though, the same analysis looked at 27 studies into spontaneous abortion and did find an increased risk of experiencing a spontaneous abortion (pregnancy loss, aka miscarriage) during early pregnancy, and a 'significantly increased' risk for those drinking between 300mg and 600mg of coffee a day. The analysis even mentioned one study that found for every additional 100mg of caffeine its participants took each day, their chances of pregnancy loss rose 14 per cent. The analysis suggested caffeine might cause higher rates of loss because it has been associated with decreased levels of both oestrogen and hCG, the pregnancy hormone, and higher levels of substances that might affect – you guessed it – blood flow to the placenta, so the acupuncturists might be right about blood flow.

Professor Tim's view? He points out that studies into coffee drinking are difficult because correlation is not causation. 'As with many things, this is difficult to study because it could be that people who drink excess caffeine do other things in life to excess, so it's very hard to disentangle lifestyle factors,' he says. But he adds that most things are generally OK in moderation. 'The most recent review studies have suggested small to moderate amounts of caffeine are not detrimental to people's fertility. I think with caffeine, as with many other things, it's about being sensible. If people are knocking back a few cups of coffee a day, it probably doesn't do any harm, but it might do, so perhaps back off or try decaffeinated coffee or tea, as it can be hard to tell the difference.'

The bottom line? 'A small to moderate amount, a couple of cups a day, isn't going to do any harm. Beyond that, just be sensible.'

Acupuncture

This is one that comes up a lot. It's almost a rite of passage for anyone going through fertility treatment to at least try acupuncture. For those uninitiated, acupuncture is an ancient Chinese medicine that involves placing very fine needles into the skin in various parts of the body to produce a therapeutic effect. Generally it goes like this: you lie on a nice treatment table, your acupuncturist lightly taps these needles into your skin and you stay lying down for around 30 minutes listening to very relaxing music. Some people fall asleep because it is very relaxing. Others (me included) go into their own little world, feeling all floaty and delicious.

It works by stimulating nerve endings (in a non-painful way), which encourages the release of endorphins. We all know about these dudes: they are the happy hormones. My acupuncturist explained that it helped to redirect energy to parts of the body that might need it. I liked this idea.

There are lots of studies into whether it can actually help fertility and increase IVF success rates, but none are particularly conclusive. Professor Tim has seen evidence that it can bring on ovulation in women with PCOS (polycystic ovary syndrome), and even though evidence for IVF success is scant, he's a fan: 'Interestingly, we undertook some research back in Oxford in the 1990s looking at acupuncture and fertility for women with PCOS, which meant that they weren't ovulating. There is some evidence that in patients with PCOS, it can help to induce ovulation. With unexplained infertility there doesn't appear to be any benefit of acupuncture in terms of increasing numbers of babies. There are loads of studies done with acupuncture and IVF, and it's fair to say that the studies are fairly conflicting. But if acupuncture helps people to feel more relaxed and in control during the IVF process, that is a positive outcome.'

Emma and I both had acupuncture. We both really enjoyed it. But neither of us could tell you whether it made any difference or not – other than to put us in a really great mood. I think it also helped that we both saw a fertility specialist; she knew all the right questions to ask and had plenty of advice for us (it was a bit like therapy in the end).

The first time I did it, I felt like I had an out-of-body experience, I definitely felt a rush of happy hormones and floated all the way home. Not everyone has this and it might not be for you, which is absolutely fine. I've heard of women hating it but doing it because they felt they should; I really don't think anyone should force themselves. If you like it and it makes you feel good, great! If not, that's cool, too. There will be other things that you might enjoy more.

Avoiding toxins

When you're looking into ways to prepare your body for fertility treatment or IVF, you'll probably come across the term BPA (or bisphenol A). In the IVF and infertility community, BPAs are a common enemy, but they are largely unheard of in the general population. I remember when I was at school, people used to tell us not to reuse the same single-use water bottles (this was a trend at the time – nothing says chic like a week-old Evian bottle with a faded saggy label). I never really understood the thinking behind this rule until I started researching infertility and chatting to the TTC community. Plastic water bottles were one of the first things to go on my list. I'll go into the others shortly, but first let's look at the science.

BPA is a chemical that, it has been suggested, messes around with your natural hormones, particularly oestrogen, testosterone and thyroid – all important players in the reproductive system. For this reason you might hear it referred to as an endocrine disruptor. It sounds like a baddie in a sci-fi movie. The aforementioned Rebecca Fett references a 2008 study by Dr Sandie Lenie that showed BPAs damage the development of eggs – creating chromosomal abnormalities as the eggs mature in the three or so months before ovulation. So far, so shit.

The biggest problem with BPAs is that they're found everywhere. From plastic food containers and tins of food to retail receipts: the modern world is a BPA minefield. It can be quite scary when you start to read into this, but the advice we have had from a number of professionals is not to panic about it. You'll never avoid BPAs completely, but you can take some small steps to reduce your exposure. The following advice can be found on the US National Institute of Environmental Health Studies site:

- Don't microwave polycarbonate plastic food containers. Polycarbonate is strong and durable, but

over time it may break down from over-use at high
temperatures.

- Plastic containers have recycle codes on the bottom.
  Some, but not all, plastics that are marked with recycle
  codes 3 or 7 may be made with BPAs.
- Reduce your use of canned foods.
- When possible, opt for glass, porcelain or stainless
  steel containers, particularly for hot food or liquids.

Emma and I stopped buying single-use water bottles and switched
to stainless steel bottles – Emma waxes lyrical about Chillies as
a brand of these; I'm brand agnostic. Tupperware fans need not
panic too much. You can replace your hard plastic containers with
glass ones – IKEA does a particularly cost-effective set.

Emma also went through a phase of trying not to touch
receipts. This is great in theory but pretty tricky in practice. Sales
staff at the till give you a pretty funny look if you refuse to touch
the receipt they brandish at you. An easier way to deal with this
is to wash your hands after you've handled them – particularly
before eating.

Phthalates

The other term you may hear bandied around in relation to
toxins is phthalates. These are another known toxin found
in everyday products. They're quite widely used in cleaning
products, fragranced cosmetics and perfume. These are also
endocrine disruptors and can mess around with your essential
reproductive hormones. These bad boys have also been found
to be bad for eggs and sperm and can cause something called
oxidative stress.

Finding out about this sent me on a bit of a mission. I certainly didn't replace all my cosmetics at once (bloody expensive trip to the shops) but I got into researching and finding phthalate-free alternatives that I liked. It all started with a trip to a giant Whole Foods – purveyor of eye-wateringly expensive nut butters and some rather lovely phthalate-free cosmetics. If you live in the UK, Holland & Barrett is a bit easier on the bank balance. I started with shampoo, conditioner, deodorant and body wash. They say that body lotion is also an important one to swap because you lather it across your whole body. Embarrassingly, I don't really use body lotion. Yes, I am as scaly as a snake. I really need to sort that out.

I also got a bit hooked on organic make-up at this point. I bought some foundation on the trip to Whole Foods and thanks to our friend Keeley Dwight, who held an organic make-up pop-up event, I also bought new concealer and lipstick. Emma never bothered with make-up. I think I went for it because I've never had great skin and I thought that if I used all organic products my skin would clear up, leaving me with the complexion of a 21-year-old Brazilian model. Full disclosure, this didn't happen, and, if I'm honest, I never did find a new foundation that worked for me, so I ended up going back to Lancôme. Keeley swears by it though, so if you're interested, I'd recommend trying a few out. I just didn't have great luck.

One thing I did stick to was giving up wearing perfume and nail varnish. These are both on the list of phthalate-filled cosmetics. But I hasten to add that I found this relatively easy. I think the key take-away from all this should hopefully be to change what you can but don't feel that you have to change everything.

Last but not least, we can't talk about detoxifying without

mentioning cleaning products. Emma and I both switched to more natural household cleaning products during our IVF journeys. As you can imagine, harsh cleaning products are full of harmful chemicals. Switching can benefit you and the environment (a tasty win-win). We found brands such as Method and Ecover quite good. A small word of warning: natural cleaning products aren't quite as effective as harsh chemical ones. You'll find yourself scrubbing for a tad longer. But hopefully you'll agree that it's worth it.

Nutrition

As we know, what you eat is a big contributing factor to your health and the way you feel. It makes sense that if you want to be in the best possible position to conceive, diet could have a part to play. That's definitely not to say that the fact you haven't been living on kale and kombucha is why you haven't got pregnant. But being as healthy as possible will give you a head start. Personally, I didn't give anything up, I simply added more of what I knew was good for me and had less of what I knew wasn't.

Eating your way to success: Melanie Brown, fertility nutritionist

'Planning your pre-conception diet can often be quite a therapeutic tool. It gives a sense of control and a feeling that you have done everything you can to help yourselves realise your goal of being a parent. And you will just feel brilliant too!

'I use the Mediterranean diet as a base, and then add all my good fertility foods to it. It's my anti-ageing diet for eggs! I eat loads of orange carotene-rich vegetables and dark green leafy cruciferous vegetables such as broccoli, berries and fish, nuts, seeds and olive oil, and plenty of protein to build up those eggs for IVF. Folate, iodine, zinc and iron, vitamin D, omega-3 fats and vitamin E are critical in foods for fertility.

'In fact, vitamin E (found in nuts, seeds and greens) is probably the most famous of all the fertility-enhancing vitamins, being made up of chemicals called tocopherols and tocotrienols. The name comes from the *Greek* "τόκος" (*tókos* meaning "birth") and "φέρειν" (*phérein*, "to bear or carry"), so tocopherol actually means "to carry a pregnancy". You couldn't have a better reason than that to eat those foods.

'And let's not forget the man. Vets and farmers know more about male fertility than anyone else. In fact, there has probably been more research done on bull and stallion sperm than human sperm because the best sperm for breeding is very valuable. The food fed to male breeding animals is the best quality and rich in nutrients. In fact, there's a famous bull in India whose owner feeds him a cocktail of vitamins to enhance his amazingly fertile sperm!

'Sometimes there is a bit of a time limit to the IVF countdown, so the eating plan might be a little more focused, and sometimes you may just be trying naturally. But couples still need to have a life: some cake or fries, a coffee, a beer or a glass of good wine – good endorphins are essential and there has to be a balance.'

A note on pineapple

Ah, the pineapple. If you're new to the world of TTC, you might have noticed a proliferation of pineapples. You'll see them in people's profile pics, worn in jewellery form, on socks worn for IVF transfers, on pencil cases used to hold medication,

T-shirts – you name it, there's a pineapple on it. Emma has a lovely gold pineapple necklace and we've both got IVF Babble pineapple pins. The exotic fruit has become the unlikely symbol of the TTC world. But why?

Well . . . the theory goes something like this: pineapple contains bromelain, which has anti-inflammatory properties. If you eat pineapple core (which contains the highest concentration of bromelain) on the day of your transfer (or after you've ovulated if you're TTCing naturally) it can help you to conceive by reducing any inflammation in the uterus and, depending who you speak to, might also increase the quantity and quality of cervical mucus.

Sounds great. Who doesn't like pineapple? Well, the core is a bit gross. But is it true? Professor Tim says it's an interesting one.

'There's quite a lot of research looking into the use of bromelain for helping wound healing. Not putting pineapples on the skin exactly but using bromelain medically. It can also affect blood clotting – it has blood thinning properties – so people on blood thinning agents need to be very careful not to drink pineapple juice.

'The question is whether pineapples actually improve fertility. I couldn't find anything published on this in any medical journal. All you can find is people's opinions on the Internet – that may or may not be correct.

'I believe the thinking is that it helps your blood flow to the uterus and encourages implantation. But it's not been shown that taking aspirin, for instance, which thins the blood, makes any difference to implantation so I'm not really sure how something such as pineapple could either.'

Popping pills – the minefield of fertility supplements

Another important piece of advice you're likely to get from your doctor/IVF clinic is to take a prenatal vitamin when you're trying to conceive. The main focus of these will be folic acid, which is critical for preventing neural tube birth defects such as spina bifida. The NHS also recommends that you consider taking something with vitamin D, too, as it's good for the baby's bone health. It has also been shown to be good for fertility and is linked with better results in IVF, so it's a thumbs up from us.

This all seems fairly straightforward, but if you start to dig into it, you'll find a range of fertility supplements, most of which contain way more ingredients than folic acid and vitamin D. Common additions to the magic mix are L-arginine, magnesium, iron, zinc, selenium and a spread of vitamin B types (1–3, 6 and 12). One of the most common conception multi-vitamins, Pregnacare, has 20 different ingredients. There are so many of these supplements out there that it's hard to know which ones are best. Some are naturally derived and therefore come with a heftier price tag.

Then, at some point, you'll come across the old folate vs folic acid debate – it's a heated one. Emma and I were talking on a panel at a fertility event one time and there was a nutritionist also speaking. She started singing the praises of folate (the natural form of synthetically created folic acid), she went as far as to tell people that they shouldn't take folic acid. There was almost a punch-up. Some audience members were rightly confused and upset, given that the NHS recommends you should take it.

The main argument for taking folate over folic acid is that some people don't process folic acid well. This is down to the MTHFR gene: an inherited gene that helps to create the protein that converts folic acid into something our bodies can use. Some people have a mutation of this gene, which results in a reduced ability to use folic acid in the way we intend it. For these people, folate is definitely preferential to folic acid. But does that mean everyone should switch?

'For the vast majority of women, there is no benefit in taking folate rather than folic acid – the only difference would be the expense,' says Professor Tim. Nutritionists will certainly argue against this, suggesting that the natural form is better. It probably depends on where you already sit on the organic sliding scale. If most of your products are already organic and naturally derived, I imagine you'll opt for folate.

Personally, I used both during my TTC journey. I used Pregnacare the majority of the time, before switching to an organic prenatal supplement by a company called Wild Nutrition while I was doing IVF. I have no idea if this had any impact other than on my bank balance. If you're wondering what to do, I would recommend reading up about it and making a decision yourself. Unless, of course, you know you have the MTHFR mutation, in which case find a supplement with folate. Emma, for the record, took folic acid the whole time – never wavering in the face of expensive alternatives.

MYTH BUSTING: Raspberry leaf tea

The myth Drinking raspberry leaf tea strengthens the uterine wall.

When I told Emma I was struggling to conceive, she asked me if I was drinking raspberry leaf tea. This was the first time I'd heard of it. I hadn't delved deeply enough into online TTC forums, clearly. Online you'll find plenty of women extolling the benefits of the herbal tea bags; the predominant reasoning being that it supports implantation by strengthening the uterine wall. I never did bother buying a box. It turns out perhaps that was for the best.

The bust: false It seems that there's no evidence of raspberry leaf tea being linked to conception. 'When I used to do obstetrics in the nineties, midwives who were pro-natural health often used raspberry leaf tea to try to induce labour,' explains Professor Tim. 'It has fallen out of fashion now, but there are some studies suggesting that it helps to stimulate uterine contractions. I checked through a huge database and couldn't find anything published about raspberry leaf teas and conception.'

It turns out that it's probably not a great idea to take while TTC because it can have an impact on you once you are pregnant. 'If taken during pregnancy, it can impact sugar levels in women, so care needs to be taken with it in pregnancy,' says Prof Tim. 'It's not a licensed drug, so taking it up until conception is fine, but once conception has occurred, people need to be careful. It does affect the uterus in pregnant women, but there are no data to suggest it improves fertility rates.'

Conclusion

We hope that this has been helpful and not too overwhelming. There is so much advice out there, and it is very difficult to work out which of it you'd like to take on board, if any. By talking you through some of the advice that's out there, we've tried to make sense of it for you. Sadly, we can't advise you on what to do with this information.

Ultimately, the best thing that you can do is listen to your doctor or clinic and take their advice. Beyond that, it's up to you. Most experts you'll speak to will just encourage you to be healthy. Everything in moderation, try to keep a healthy weight – look after yourself. No one can argue with that.

3

How to Lose Friends and Alienate People

(Emma)

Trying unsuccessfully for a baby is a deeply isolating process. Because it's such a fundamental part of the human experience, it's a rare person who doesn't have something to say about it, and those opinions are almost always deeply unhelpful.

What's kind of wonderful is that crap comments from friends and relatives unite everyone who is TTC. Whoever you are, the 'just relax' and 'at least' brigades will be on hand to make the process that little bit more frustrating. We've had listeners from every age, nationality, race, gender and religion, single people, people in same-sex relationships and straight couples and they have told us that their friends and family have said roughly the same mildly offensive things.

I blame the taboo surrounding TTC. For a very long time we heard only about people's success stories: 'I tried for years for a baby, and now I have one!' It's only very recently that people have started openly talking about how much they are struggling. Because of this long history of hiding our experiences, people assume that if you try hard enough, you'll eventually be success-ful. 'Just relax' and 'my friend was about to do IVF and then got pregnant on holiday' becomes an easy way out of a conversation that could be about to get very uncomfortable (and, gasp, emo-tional) for the person talking to you.

In this chapter I'll cover how to react to those comments, but also how to deal with your friends getting pregnant when you can't (and the crap comments *they* make as well). We'll also both share stories about terrible friendship moments during our TTC process.

What you'll find in this chapter:

- Why your friends don't get it.
- Why people make those comments.
- How to educate others.
- How to deal with pregnancy announcements.
- How to help your friends to help you.
- Building your TTC support network.
- Good responses to crap comments.

My story

My best friend is called Sophie. We practically grew up together. During senior school, we were at each other's houses almost every weekend. We shared a wardrobe, deep and passionate loves for Thom Yorke and too much eyeliner, and we both learned to play the opening bars of 'Everybody Hurts' by R.E.M. on the guitar to impress boys. Our first kisses were with the same boy, a week apart, then, years later, we were each other's maids of honour as we got married in the same year, a few months apart (different boys this time, to be clear).

Sophie waited until after my wedding to start trying for a baby, because she is considerate like that, and also because I had really, really good wine at my reception. But within three months of my big day, she was pregnant. Almost a year to the day later, her beautiful little girl was born – and I started trying for my own baby. That's when things started to get weird.

While Sophie was coping with the intensity of emotion that comes from becoming a mum for the first time, I was experiencing the rollercoaster of ups and downs that is trying for a baby.

As the months passed, my thoughts towards pregnant women and mums turned increasingly bitter. One day, I sent a text message to Sophie explaining how much I had wanted to punch a pregnant woman as I walked past her. She didn't reply. The next day, I told her I hadn't given up my seat on the Tube when a pregnant woman got on. She didn't reply again. The day after that, she sent me a long Facebook message essentially telling me to sort my shit out, and that she felt she couldn't share anything about her daughter with me because she didn't want me directing those bitter thoughts towards her.

I got upset. She got upset. We didn't speak for a week. Then we had a tearful reunion and I realised that sharing every single horrible, vitriolic thought I was having probably hadn't been a great idea, even though we had always shared everything before. Meanwhile, she had spoken to a friend who'd been through IVF, who helped her to understand the stress people struggling with infertility can experience.

That incident is the only proper argument we have ever had (except one about a boy who drove a Morris Minor, but that wasn't really a *proper* argument), but it's also a highly convenient illustration of how even the most joined-at-the-hip friendships can suffer when infertility strikes.

Why don't my friends get it?

Most of our friendships arise out of shared experience. You meet people at school or university or work, and then you go through the same big life events together at roughly the same time: graduation, relationships, promotions, that unfortunate fake-tan phase. It's why, for several summers in your late twenties and early thirties, it feels like you're spending your entire disposable income on attending increasingly pricey weddings, because everyone does the same things at once. It's why we choose, or stick with, the friends we do.

Then it reaches a certain point, and the strike-addled train operator of life does a strange thing. While some of your friends are at the 'Single and Loving It' station, partying on the platform and batting their eyelashes at handsome strangers, others go straight to 'Popping out Babies Junction', exhausted and covered in puke, admittedly, but hanging out with a whole bunch of similarly tired, similarly vom-soaked people.

If you're going through infertility, it feels as if there's been a signal failure. You're stuck on a train between the two stations, desperately trying to tell your friends when you're due to arrive, but the driver isn't giving you much information. It's heartbreaking, but it's also frustrating as hell. Suddenly, your paths have diverged and your shared experiences feel like they're slipping away.

Even the best friends won't necessarily understand what you're experiencing when you're going through infertility. The cycle of hope, grief, hope again can be difficult to articulate, and because there's no one 'event' you can point to – 'this thing happened to me: I am sad' – people find it hard to understand what you're upset about.

Even if you have experienced pregnancy loss, society's view of fertility – that it's something you can switch off and on again, that you can always 'get back on the horse' – means that people's sympathy can be limited, which is not what you need when you're going through a traumatic experience.

Why friends and family react like that

The fact that there is no one event you can pinpoint as 'the awful thing' immediately separates it from most of life's most difficult experiences: loss, diagnosis of a terrible illness, redundancy, divorce. To some people, even pregnancy loss doesn't always 'count'; after all, it wasn't a person you met, was it? And you can always get pregnant again.

Playing catch-up

It might sound ridiculous, but those of us going through infertility need to have compassion for our friends. Stay with me: what you need to understand is that all those idiotic clichés they come out with, which we'll come to later, come from a place of love. Yes, even 'just relax'.

The first thing to understand is that your friends are playing catch-up. You've already been through months of not conceiving or baby loss, you've googled everything under the sun and you've been using raspberry leaf tea, sperm-friendly lube and enough supplements to make you rattle for *months*.

Your friends, on the other hand, haven't spent hours trawling through forum posts or discussing the most effective sex positions with strangers on Instagram at 3am. They're new to this, so of course they'll ask you whether you've tried booking a holiday because their friend's cousin did that and that's how they got pregnant. It's exactly what you thought nine months ago when you first realised that things weren't working. You still have the tan lines to prove it.

Realising they're just not up to speed helps to take the pressure off and remove some of the anger. Of course, it's not your job to help them catch up, but if you feel their support would help you, it might be worth trying. There's actually a very straightforward way to demonstrate the pain you're going through, says Tracey Sainsbury, a fertility counsellor and the co-author of *Making Friends With Your Fertility*: show your friends that little clip from the Pixar movie *Up*. You know the one: the elderly widower reminisces about his and his wife's life together, and their struggles to have a child. If you need a good cry, go and watch it now. I'll wait.

Say to your friends: 'This is what we're going through. We don't know what's going to happen, but I need the same compassion as how this film makes you feel.'

'Sometimes we need a robust shield of resilience to recognise our friends are playing catch-up and to do everything we can to help them understand so they're not floundering,' says Tracey. 'Let them know: "Look, it's OK, I'm going to be all over the place, I just need you to listen and give me a cuddle. Don't try to fix it because you can't."'

Frame of reference

Another reason friends and family have trouble empathising with your struggle is that although we might insist we are generous souls, the way we respond to other people's suffering is through our own frame of reference, says Tracey. It's why Brexit divided the country so much: young Remainer and his Uncle Leaver couldn't get out of their own heads and into each other's.

In other words, your friends have put you in a box, and news like 'I can't conceive' will cause them to either freak out that this might also become their experience, or feel profoundly guilty that it's not. Either way, this is about them, not you. Your friends want you to fit their mould. It sounds selfish, but it's how humans have learned to relate to one another. And besides, it's partly because they love you so much.

Tracey: 'If your friend puts you on a pedestal as the perfect couple and assumes that you'd just conceive naturally, it can be a shock. If you're similar in terms of age or build or levels of healthiness, there can be a fear – oh my goodness you're having problems, am I going to have problems, too? And if they've got children, there can be that shame or embarrassment – "I don't know what to say."'

The key is making it clear that nothing they can say will make things better. The easiest thing to try is: 'I need you to be comfortable with my sadness.' Simple, straightforward, to the point.

Show, don't tell: Easy ways to help your friends understand

Netflix A recent push in infertility-related content means movies such as *Only You, Private Life, One More Shot, Vegas Baby!* and one series of *Master of None* give an insight into the highs and lows surrounding infertility and its treatment.

Fertility Network UK The UK's fertility charity produces a fact sheet to help friends and family understand how to approach those struggling to conceive.

Podcasts A lot of our listeners have told us that sharing BFN with friends and family has helped them to empathise with what they're going through. Other podcasts – such as The Long Road to Baby, Infertile AF, The Fertility Podcast and the brilliant Matt and Doree's Eggcellent Adventure – are available (but ours is better).

Celebrities Michelle Obama's decision to discuss her struggle with infertility has opened the doors to other celebrities admitting they, too, have been through it (yes, that actress who conceived twins aged 50 didn't do it naturally. It's a shock, I know), while the harrowing photos Chrissy Teigen posted of the birth of her stillborn son, Jack, opened many people's eyes to the pain of pregnancy and baby loss. Sharing these stories with your friends and family might help them to understand what you're experiencing.

Things people will say to you and how you might respond

When people don't really understand what's happening to a loved one, their instinct is usually to try to solve their problems. That means you'll probably hear the same lines, over and over again. Here are some suggested ways to respond:

The line 'Just relax!'

The old classic. Everyone, including (at the beginning, before you punch him/her in the face) your partner, will try it. The idea is that simply by unclenching, you will magically become pregnant.

The response: 'I *am* relaxed, but I'm also arming myself with information and I'm talking about my experience – that doesn't mean I'm stressed out.'

People see 'just relax' as helpful. They don't want you to worry – and of course they've heard the classic cliché about someone who couldn't get pregnant, stopped thinking about it, went on a holiday, got drunk and *boom!* got pregnant, so they tell you, because that's the only thing they can think to do.

You could try to explain that by doing your research and arming yourself with information, you are simply taking some control over your own fertility, which is only going to increase your chances. Information is power. And just because you're telling them about it does not mean that you are unrelaxed. It doesn't mean you're stressed. You're just informed.

And although I said earlier in the chapter that people are coming from a place of love with these reactions it's also an indication of just how much further feminism has to go. God forbid a woman would think about and want to take control of her own fertility rather than just sitting around, swooning occasionally and waiting for the magical forces of nature to bless her with a child. Very occasionally, it's just straightfor-ward victim blaming: that person is telling you your infertility is *your fault* when it almost definitely isn't.

The line 'So when are you having kids? The clock's ticking . . .'

Another absolute classic, this is usually said by older relatives who like to see lots of children around and want to see the family line being carried on, or during really awkward conversations at parties when the speakers can't really think of anything else to say.

The response: 'We've been trying for three years and I've done x, y and z. Got any tips?'

A lot of how you respond to this old chestnut is related to how comfortable you are discussing your own fertility. It's perfectly reasonable to brush it off with a classic, vague, 'Ah, we're thinking about it.' If you're more comfortable talking about what you're going through, though, there's nothing wrong with being honest: 'Actually I've been trying for three years.' Then, if that person has upset you, you could always add in an extra: 'I can tell you all about my cervical mucus quality if you're interested.' The fact is, no one has the right to discuss what you do or don't choose to do with your body. The decisions you, or you and your partner, make is your business.

The line 'Have you tried acupuncture?'

This was a particularly irritating one for me. Westerners tend to turn to complementary medicine when conventional doctors are at a loss as to what to do next. We've both met dozens of women who swear it was the only reason little Ottilie is here at all.

The response: 'Does everyone do that before they get pregnant, then?'

Look, we've talked about the benefits of acupuncture, but if you don't like the idea of lying still for an hour while dozens of tiny needles are stuck in you, the benefits you're likely to derive from it are minimal. The fact is, most people who get pregnant do so just fine without any of the crazy stuff infertile people try. In lots of cases, people keep drinking and smoking until worryingly late into their pregnancy. Although studies have suggested acupuncture can have benefits (I certainly found it helped me to feel calm during one of the most horrible times of my life) those studies aren't conclusive enough to be worth making yourself miserable for. Other treatments – acupressure, for instance – can also have beneficial effects, so can an evening of wine and Netflix.

The line 'You probably won't need IVF. My friend got pregnant when she was just about to start'

This is a confusing one: either the world is littered with women who got knocked up on the brink of doing IVF but they're all hiding from us, or it happened to one woman and she just has a lot of friends. Either way, that kind of comment isn't helpful.

The response: 'It's unlikely that will happen to me.'

'Infertility' is a catch-all term that covers everything from mechanical problems (blocked tubes and fibroids) to chronic illness (endometriosis and PCOS) to the whole umbrella of male-factor infertility. Their friend might have had a miracle pregnancy because they had changed their diet or started taking certain supplements to help them with their difficulty, but that doesn't mean it'll happen for you.

The line 'Well you can just adopt. There are plenty of kids out there who need a new home'

The word 'just' should be punishable by law. Anyone going through infertility realises 'just' anything – doing IVF, adopting, finding a surrogate – is a long and emotional ride. No one 'just' does anything.

The response: 'We may explore that at some stage, but for now I am trying to come to terms with my grief.'

Here's the thing: back in the day, when abortion was illegal, single mothers were routinely shamed, and flame-haired orphans sang about hard-knock lives, people regularly gave up their new-borns for adoption. But times have, thankfully, changed, and every effort is made to keep children with their families before they are put into care.

To ensure the children who *are* taken into care are matched with the right families, adoption involves lengthy and invasive checks before you've even been matched with a child, then months, or even years, of waiting to find the right little person. All of which is a way of saying that although adoption can be a rewarding way to complete your family, no one has ever 'just' adopted.

The line 'At least you know you can get pregnant/the miscarriage was early'

This is perhaps the most hurtful thing a person can say to some-one who has just experienced pregnancy loss, who is grieving the loss of their longed-for baby.

The response: 'My baby died.'

It doesn't matter what stage you lost your baby at, it's likely you had already imagined its future in great detail. If you're any-thing like us, you had worked out your due date, you had started thinking about NCT classes, you'd casually looked up nurseries in your local area and you had vaguely wondered what university it might go to. In other words, you are a parent who has lost a child. I'll talk about this in detail in the chapter on pregnancy loss, but for now, know this: your grief should be treated like everyone else's, not casually brushed off.

Pregnancy announcements and dealing with social occasions

It's the moment anyone going through infertility dreads. It's Tabitha's birthday. You're having dinner. Your fertility radar sounds an emergency alarm: she isn't drinking. After the start-ers, she smiles beatifically and exchanges looks with Mr Tabitha. He rubs her back. She sighs. 'So, we've got some news', she says. Mr Tabitha looks smug. Your stomach lurches.

The happy news is announced. 'And we weren't even trying!' they beam. You make an excuse and run to the loo. You lock yourself in a stall and cry, then after a while you text your friend/partner to tell them that you're leaving, because you're not giving bloody Tabitha the satisfaction of seeing you like this, especially not after she got that promotion last week and you didn't.

Just to emphasise how much *everyone has to put up with this,* here's Gabby's experience:

Gabby's story

I was out with friends one Sunday having a roast. One of them approached the table with a Bloody Mary and when my husband exclaimed that it was a marvellous idea, she awkwardly said, 'It's a Virgin Mary, actually. *I'm pregnant. I'm sorry!*' Cue a very awkward couple of seconds, until we both snapped out of it and said, 'Wow, congratulations!' with all the energy we could muster. I wanted the ground to swallow me. I wanted to disappear in a cloud of smoke (if only people still lit up Marlboros in pubs).

As it turned out, everyone knew except us. She had agonised about how to tell us, not got around to it, and then, *boom!*, it came out all wrong over a Bloody Shame (bartender lingo for spicy tomato juice). We stayed for the roast chicken and left shortly afterwards. I felt sick. I felt like everyone was watching for my reaction. And even though they were probably just eyeing up my Yorkshire pudding, I decided I wanted out.

This is never a good way to find out that your friend is pregnant. It's uncomfortable for everyone involved. But once the moment had passed, I was fine about her pregnancy. Nay! Delighted for her. It's the moment of finding out that is hard. That's the bit that hurts.

Why you feel like this

This is arguably the most horrible part of infertility: finding it difficult to be happy when something amazing happens for the people around you. People experience this differently: whereas some are able to separate being happy for others from feeling sad for themselves, I am part of the other group: all bitterness, all the time.

The first thing to say is that *these feelings are natural*. You are not a horrible person for having them. It seems so unfair when others are able to achieve the one thing you want most in the world, sometimes by accident.

One way of looking at it is this: parenthood is not an easy ride. You won't sleep. Having a shower by yourself will become a luxury. You will, at some point, get another human being's faeces in your hair. And if you're struggling to conceive, it feels like just getting to the point where you can cheerfully massage shit into your scalp is going to be a very long, very boring process.

Therefore, the strength of the envy we experience when someone else makes a pregnancy announcement is simply your brain reminding you that it's still up for this. It's a little opportunity to check with yourself that you're prepared for the hardships you're about to endure.

What's important to recognise is that, right now, you are the one experiencing pain. The World Health Organization (WHO) classifies infertility as 'leading to disability', so treat yourself like someone who is sick: do not attend Tabitha's baby shower if you can't face it. Leave the restaurant and text Tabitha later to explain what happened.

This is applicable in any situation where kids and/or large quantities of pregnant women might be present: christenings, first birthday parties, any afternoon tea. Make an excuse, any excuse, and then *don't beat yourself up about it later*. Tabitha will live, particularly if you explain your predicament to her (although a simple 'I had to leave' has the benefit of making you seem aloof and mysterious).

How friends can make pregnancy announcements easier for you

Just before Sophie started trying for her second baby (and, as it turned out, third baby – for yes, they were twins), we went on holiday to Paris together. During that weekend we ate a lot of steak, drank a lot of champagne and talked for three solid days. As we hurtled past the Arc de Triomphe in what might very well have been an unlicensed Uber, Sophie admitted that she was planning to start trying again after we got back.

We talked about how she would share her news and decided the best thing to do would be a brief phone call. Which is why, *exactly four weeks later* when I noticed I had several dozen missed calls from her, I knew what it was going to be about.

'This is the call,' she said.

'OK. Congratulations,' I said.

'We've been friends for 20 years. If you need to take the next nine months off, I'm OK with that,' she said. 'I'm going to go now.' That might very well be the kindest thing anyone has said to me during this entire shitshow. But as it turned out, I was able to be happy for her.

It's also worth pointing out that as time has passed and I have become more public about my infertility, friends have become increasingly thoughtful about how they have told me they're pregnant. Instead of the big announcement, they've messaged me first or had a quiet word – because forewarned is forearmed.

How to prepare your friends

Obviously, telling your friends what you're going through might not be the easiest thing to do (definitely best not to do it just after she's shared her news). But laying the groundwork among close friends can help. If they know you're having trouble, they can be understanding when you don't show up to social occasions. Lunches, drinks, birthdays, group holidays – we've missed them all over the years we've been trying for babies, but because our friends knew what was going on, they were able to empathise, rather than be angry.

Being able to explain what is happening to your friends means that even when a code red hits and someone announces that they are pregnant, they will be able to do it sensitively. The more people understand what you are going through, the more they can help you go through it.

Here are some ideas:

Pre-warning The easiest way to hear the news of a friend's impending pregnancy is *before* the big 'surprise!' moment in front of your entire group of friends. It means that you are ready to arrange your face in a way that says 'congratulations' when all you're thinking is: *Why isn't this me?* Admittedly, it isn't easy to casually drop this into conversation, but if you can find a way to explain to friends-who-might-be-trying that a heads-up ahead of the big announcement will help you to process their news properly, it will help you out in the long term.

WhatsApp doc? As your fertility jourrrney (*sorry*) progresses, your friends will naturally want to show they care by checking in with you. Sometimes, just admitting that things haven't worked out is too hard. Some couples create a WhatsApp group for those close to them, so that they can provide updates on their treatments (and emotional states). If it all gets too much, you can leave the group and ask your partner to provide updates. Then, when you're feeling more resilient, rejoin.

Have the conversation This can be the hardest thing to do but the most effective. One of the things we've found is that when friends get pregnant, they feel very awkward and anxious about how to tell you. This sensitive conversation early on can solve this and make finding out easier. Tell them how you want to find out so that they know what to do. Do you want to find out first? Do you want them to tell you via email so that those two blue ticks or seen notifications don't make you feel you need to react immediately?

Building your support network

One rainy Saturday in October 2018, a doctor broke the news to me that we weren't going ahead with a third round of IVF because my body had let me down yet again. As I sank into a chair in the waiting room, my phone buzzed: 'Are you OK?' A few seconds later, it buzzed again: 'What's happening?' Those weren't my closest friends. They were strangers I met on the Internet.

Support can come from anywhere, but nothing beats the empathy you'll get from those who know exactly what you're going through. There are lots of places you can turn to: your clinic may have information about a local support group, while Fertility Network UK lists meet-ups in every part of the UK.

For us, though, it was all about social media. Instagram may be known as a way for people to put a glossy filter over their lives, but Infertility Instagram is different. We started our Instagram accounts in the summer of 2018, shortly after we decided to start BFN, and within months we had a solid group of people to whom we could turn whenever things went wrong.

The best thing about social media is that it's normal women behind those accounts: they make jokes about the awkwardness of self-injecting, they laugh at strangers' reactions when they give honest answers to the question 'Why don't you have kids yet?' and they worry about what to wear when their ovaries are so swollen with hormones that wearing anything that presses against their abdomen actually hurts.

They helped me in innumerable ways: they knew what to do when my lining was too thin, they explained the confusing jargon my consultants used and they were there for me when cycles were cancelled. Whatever I was going through, there was someone else who had been there. If you've chosen not to tell anyone about your infertility, you can create an anonymous account – providing an instant support group when you need it the most.

How to build your TTC social media account

Remain anonymous If, like many people, you'd like to remain anonymous on your TTC Instagram account, use a different email from your other account (if you have one). Otherwise, people who follow your 'civilian' account will get served your TTC one as a suggestion.

Follow the right people Any community has its leaders. Find them and you'll discover the rest of the community.

Hashtags Yes, they're quite cringe, but using hashtags such as #ttccommunity, #ttcjourney and #infertilitysupport will help other people find you.

Contribute If you have experience or knowledge of something another person is going through, drop them a line to let them know. The community is all about sharing your expertise, so make sure you give as well as take.

Conclusion

One of the most fundamentally difficult parts of infertility is what it does to our relationships – people we were once closest to suddenly feel very distant. The feeling of isolation can be incredibly painful.

Part of the tragedy of it, though, is that you're *not* alone. I've said it a lot already, but I'll say it again: one in six couples are going through this. Your friends may not get it, your family may not get it, but there are people out there who do. Your job is to find them.

The taboo *is* lifting, albeit slowly, meaning that an increasing number of people are beginning to share their experiences with their friends and family. Having that conversation can be difficult, and the reactions when you do share can sometimes leave you feeling even more alone. But if you can find even one person who responds with empathy, that will make your 'jourrrney' a lot easier. Plus, you might find that once you start sharing, others will start to tell you about their experiences.

If you don't feel comfortable doing that yet, that's fine: find your space – whether that's an anonymous social media account or even a therapist's couch – and share there instead. Just find somewhere you can open up.

4

Getting a Diagnosis

(Emma)

There are many routes to realising that something isn't quite right. Perhaps you're a 'type A' personality who has been trying for six months and doesn't want to take the risk of waiting any longer; perhaps you've experienced a pregnancy loss – or a few – and you're scared of what happens when you next see two lines on your pregnancy test. Perhaps you weren't even actively TTC, and you just said you would 'see what happens', but a few months (or even years) on you aren't feeling quite so chilled any more. Perhaps you've already had a child and are struggling to conceive your second. Whatever stage you're at, your first step will be a conversation with your GP.

In the UK, NICE guidelines state that people should seek testing after a year of trying to conceive, although anyone who is concerned about delays in conception should be offered an initial assessment, at which point your GP will offer you some 'helpful' tips about your lifestyle, ask about your sexual history and, hopefully, get the ball rolling on tests.

Don't be afraid of seeing your doctor before that initial year is up: there are dozens of reasons your GP could begin investigations early, and most doctors will want to get started, so, if you need it, they can make a referral to a fertility clinic as soon as that year is up.

Still, if you think just TTC has involved a lot of waiting, you're in for a treat when it comes to the diagnosis of fertility problems. Welcome to the world's most frustrating waiting room. We recommend taking up a hobby.

What you'll find in this chapter:

- What to expect at your first GP appointment.
- Questions to ask your GP.
- Initial tests – what you will be referred for and the results you're after.
- What can go wrong – common reasons you might not be conceiving.
- Secondary infertility.
- Unexplained infertility: what is it and what does it mean?

My story

I am blessed with a naturally pessimistic streak, which means that I suspected fairly early on that things weren't going right. I finally caved and visited my GP when I was roughly nine months into trying for a baby. I was lucky to have a young, female GP who listened attentively, took me seriously and handed me tissues to clean up my eye make-up afterwards. She was also wearing a lovely tea dress – obviously not an essential detail, but it did lend the process a certain Hollywood glamour.

The questions she asked me were pretty straightforward: did I or my husband smoke? (Not unless we were having an *extremely* nice evening.) How much did we drink? (Probably too much, but we were having a hard time, OK?) Had we ever had any STIs? (Not to our knowledge.) What were our BMIs like? (Fine.) What were my periods like? (Irregular, painful and heavy.) How often were we having sex? (We were at it like desperate, miserable, robotic rabbits.)

She immediately referred us both for the first round of testing. Some happened quickly – I was able to book the blood tests that cycle – whereas others, like my pelvic ultrasound (which, by the way, is internal: don't wear a jumpsuit that day), involved waiting lists. Mr Emma trotted off to provide his sample on his day off work (a bad day, as it turned out; he assures me that providing a sperm sample isn't at all easy on a day that's 30 degrees outside and a pair of nurses is gossiping about the Olympic volleyball directly outside the room).

After all those tests came back OK, the GP referred me to our local hospital's gynaecology clinic, where they moved on to the next round of tests, a hysterosalpingogram (HSG) followed by a laparoscopy, which is where I was diagnosed with blocked tubes. Those tests took a little longer, with a 12-week waiting list for each.

What to expect at your first appointment with your GP

Katherine Richards is a GP in West London who completed a diploma in obstetrics and gynaecology. In other words: she knows her female reproductive systems. She says that NICE guidelines on fertility make the process of referring a patient 'very straightforward'. 'Fertility is something we have to deal with, unfortunately, quite a lot,' she says, which means that your GP should hopefully be well versed in the process.

The first thing your doctor should do is ask about you and your partner's lifestyle. They'll want to know how much you drink and smoke, how much stress you're under, what your diet is like and what sort of exercise you do. They'll ask about your sex life: how often you do it and how long you've been trying (bear in mind that NICE guidelines suggest every two to three days, as explained on page 10), and if there are any previous pregnancies or children that either of you have had.

They'll ask about your general and sexual health, past and present (STIs such as chlamydia can contribute to infertility), what medication you are on, what type of contraception you previously used and how long it's been since you came off it. They might then do a physical examination on one or both of you, to check for infection or physical issues.

Although you're not technically deemed to be having trouble conceiving until the one-year mark, there are lots of reasons GPs can begin investigations earlier, says Katherine. If you're over 36, you can start after six months of trying. If you or your partner has had an STI, or even if you have heavy or painful periods, that's a reason to begin tests. Just make sure you flag it in order to give your GP a good reason to get started.

She says that she'd rather begin investigations as soon as possible. 'If the first semen sample is mildly wrong, then you have to wait three months to do another sample, which is an awfully long time,' she says. And, as we all know, when it comes to fertility, time is of the essence.

To make things easier for your GP, make sure that both of

you are registered at the same surgery. If you're not, that's not a problem: it might just be a slower process. If one of you has a pre-existing condition that might affect fertility, like Mr Emma's Robertsonian translocation, go to your doctor as soon as possible (ideally before you begin TTC so that they can get the ball rolling on testing).

The doctor's grilling might be exhausting, but you'll have questions of your own. Here's what we suggest you ask:

- What's our CCG's (Clinical Commissioning Group: your local NHS funding body) policy on fertility treatment?
- How long is the waiting list for fertility treatment?
- How long are the waiting lists for tests?
- What tests are you referring me for?
- What happens if the results are borderline?
- Where will I need to go to have my tests done?
- Are there any tests that you aren't referring me for, and why not?

It's worth pointing out here that there is nothing wrong with being pushy (as long as you're polite). Although some GPs are very clued-up on fertility issues, others are more of the 'just relax' school of doctoring, which is not helpful. If they're being unyielding, you can always make an appointment with a different GP. It might also help you to have read up on the NICE recommendations. Just search 'NICE guidelines infertility'. It's not the most engaging read, but it will mean you are absolutely clear on what the rules are before you speak to your doctor.

One final note: Katherine says that in many cases you might just have to wait out the full year. 'There may not be anything else you can do,' she says. It's also worth pointing out, though, that your GP should be able to explain why they aren't referring you for tests yet. 'If you really think from what you've read that you deserve to be referred and they're not giving you a straight answer about why you can't be, there's a miscommunication.'

You deserve fertility investigations, even if . . .

We hear from a lot of podcast listeners who have either been told that they aren't entitled to fertility tests or they believe they aren't because of something they have done in the past. Nope. You deserve to find out why you aren't conceiving, even if:

- You are over 40.
- You have previously had a pregnancy loss.
- You have previously terminated a pregnancy.
- You already have a child.
- Your BMI is considered high.
- You have previously had an STI.
- You insisted you didn't want kids when you were younger (hi Emma).
- You are on any kind of medication.
- You have a history of mental health issues such as depression or an eating disorder.
- You don't think you deserve a baby.

Taking things further

First things first: we need to find out why you're not conceiving.

Initial tests: what your GP might ask for and the results you want

Your GP might refer you for the following tests:

Semen analysis This will not only test for sperm count but also for motility and morphology (how well they move and what sort of shape they are). Results-wise, you're looking for a count of at least 15 million sperm per ml (millilitre), with 39 million sperm per ejaculate or more. Progressive motility (that is, those moving forward) should be at least 32 per cent with total motility of 40 per cent (that is, including those that are moving but not going anywhere); and normal morphology (the shape) should be 4 per cent or more. Note that this means up to 96 per cent of sperm can have an abnormal shape, and this is a normal result, which is why morphology is seen by some as not very predictive of problems with fertility. If any results are abnormal, a second test should be offered, although some experts suggest a second test should be done anyway, so it might be worth pushing for that if the results are borderline.

Day 21 progesterone test Progesterone is one of the signs that you are ovulating. NICE recommends a test seven days before your next period (that is, day 21 of a 28-day cycle) or, if your cycles are irregular, a test later in your cycle (for example, day 28 of a 35-day cycle), which could be repeated each week until your period. You are looking for a result of over 15–30nmol/L (nanomoles per litre) depending on the lab and your clinic's criteria. If levels are low, check that the test was done seven days or so before your period. The greater the difference from seven days the lower the progesterone result might be even though ovulation did occur.

Ovarian reserve This usually takes the form of blood tests that measure either the level of anti-Müllerian hormone (AMH) or follicle stimulating hormone (FSH), or both. Many GPs will not have access to AMH testing. AMH can be tested on any day of the menstrual cycle with the normal range dependent on your age. AMH levels drop as your ovarian reserve reduces, which means a higher result is better. You are looking for a level of at least 5pmol/l (picomoles per litre) or so (but the result sheet will have your personal normal range on, so take a look). FSH has to be taken at the start of the cycle, around days two to five. As ovarian reserve reduces, the FSH level goes up, so a low result is better (the opposite to AMH!). You're after a number in single figures. Importantly, ovarian-reserve tests don't tell you why you're not getting pregnant. If you're having regular cycles, it makes no difference to the chance of natural conception whether you have a high or low ovarian reserve. Having a low ovarian reserve can, however, be a problem for IVF treatment, which is why NICE suggests that these tests are done only at that point for most women.

Date with Wanda (otherwise known as an internal scan) This takes the form of an ultrasound using a dildo-shaped probe, which is lubed up and inserted into your vagina (it isn't uncomfortable in the slightest, but it is most definitely a strange sensation). The person scanning you might look for two things:

firstly, the number of antral, or resting, follicles you have, which helps to establish your ovarian reserve. Secondly, it might flag up any physical problems with your uterus, such as fibroids or other abnormalities.

HSG or HyCoSy During this procedure, a technician will put a catheter through your cervix and insert dye into it. The idea is that the dye then fills your uterus and drifts up through your Fallopian tubes to demonstrate their 'patency' (that is, how clear they are). Spoiler: it isn't an especially comfortable procedure, so make sure you pop a couple of painkillers an hour or so before your appointment. (Note that the only difference between the HSG and the HyCoSy is how they see what's going on: HSG uses X-rays; HyCoSy uses ultrasound. It's also known as a fill 'n' spill test, which makes it sound a lot more fun than it is.)

Tips on taking control

Your GP should routinely show you the results of your tests, even if they appear to be within the normal ranges, but if they're anything like ours, he or she may just say 'It looks fine', and move on. This is why it's imperative that you request copies of your results. We've heard of cases where the GP has read the results wrongly (one of our podcast guests' doctors confidently assured him that his test showed a relatively healthy six million sperm: it was actually a very concerning six sperm), while for others a borderline result is actually quite worrying.

Even if the results show that you're absolutely fine, having copies of your test results to hand will mean a lot less work if, for instance, you decide to approach a private fertility clinic.

Here are some ideas to help you feel as in control as possible:

1   Buy yourself a nice, big, shiny folder, already loaded with clear pockets, then use it to file every single test result, piece of correspondence and any notes from appointments. Start at the back and work your way forward – that way you have your most recent correspondence at the start of the folder.

2   Test results are generally available from GPs two to three weeks after a blood test or procedure, although you should check how long it's likely to be at the time of your test. GPs don't habitually call you unless there is something wrong, so make a note in your diary to call them for your results a month or so after your test. Even if the results are OK, it'll be helpful to have a copy of them.

3   If you just get a short 'everything's fine', request a proper printout of your results and ask your GP to explain what everything means. If your results are borderline, it might be worth asking for a second opinion.

4   Take your fertility folder with you to *every appointment*. Computer systems used by surgeries and clinics – particularly NHS ones – are notoriously clunky, so having copies of all your test results will force your doctor to address you, rather than spend half the time trying to navigate your medical history on a screen.

5   Other information, such as a list showing the lengths of your last few cycles, might be helpful too. My carefully

prepared spreadsheet of three years of cycles (complete with colour coding based on cycle length) helped my fertility specialist to decide which drugs protocol to use during my IVF cycles.

6   If you have been referred for treatment but haven't heard back, don't just sit and wait for it to happen. Calling your GP, hospital or clinic and finding out what's going on won't threaten your place on the waiting list, but it might give you the information you need.

7   If you have been referred for treatment under a certain consultant, find out the name and number of their secretary, and speak to them – nicely. These super-organised men and women spend their days wrangling their bosses' diaries and dealing with requests from patients, so if there is a way to get higher up the waiting list they will know and you want to be at the forefront of their mind should an opportunity arise. A compliment or an empathetic comment ('I honestly don't know how you do this') can go a *very* long way. Many consultants work privately as well as for the NHS, and have secretaries for both practices, so if you're having trouble getting hold of one, try the other.

8   We're big advocates for recording appointments so that you can listen back if you find all the information overwhelming. There are even apps, such as Otter, which can automatically transcribe everything that's said (although the results are sometimes slightly questionable, particularly if you're using a lot of medical vocab).

Obviously, ask your doctor first, and if they would rather you didn't, have a notepad to hand so that you can write everything down instead.

What can go wrong

We'll tackle most of the things that can prevent you from getting pregnant or maintaining a pregnancy in more detail later in the book, but here's a quick summary of the NHS guidelines around infertility:

In women

1   **Ovulation, or lack thereof** Lack of ovulation can be caused by factors including polycystic ovary syndrome (PCOS), premature ovarian failure (also known as early menopause), or problems with your thyroid. You'll know that you aren't ovulating regularly if your periods tend to be unpredictable. Periods are late because ovulation is late, in other words the follicular phase can expand and contract, but the luteal phase tends to stay the same.

2   **Physical factors** Common physical impediments that prevent pregnancy include scarring from: abdominal surgery (to pluck an example out of thin air, my appendix surgery), which can block the Fallopian tubes or leave scars on the uterus (this is known as Asherman's syndrome); small growths around the womb called fibroids; endometriosis, where pieces of the womb lining

grow outside the womb (often causing excruciating period pains) or pelvic inflammation, which is often caused by STDs and can create scarring.

3   **Other uterine abnormalities** Some women are born with 'abnormally' shaped wombs. According to Tommy's, the pregnancy charity, a bicornuate or 'heart-shaped' uterus (definitely not as sweet as it sounds) can give you a slightly higher chance of miscarrying or having a pre-term birth, whereas a unicornuate uterus (where one side fails to develop) carries a higher risk of ectopic pregnancy, late miscarriage or pre-term birth. Septate or subseptate wombs, which have a sort of 'septum' down the middle, are associated with difficulties conceiving, plus first-trimester miscarriage and pre-term birth. Finally, there's the arcuate womb, which has a sort of dip at the top. It may very slightly increase your risk of miscarriage in the second trimester. These abnormalities are difficult to diagnose without detailed scans, or an HSG or exploratory surgery (laparoscopy or hysteroscopy), but it's worth knowing that they are a possibility, particularly if you have had a few losses and don't have an explanation for them.

4   **Drugs** We're loathe to say this, as many people depend on drugs to keep them alive or feeling OK, but it's worth a conversation with your doctor if you are on some antipsychotics, a fluid retention drug called spironolactone, or taking ibuprofen or aspirin long term. Chemotherapy can also have an effect on your fertility, although doctors should address this before treatment

begins. Obviously, doing illegal drugs is also a very bad idea when you are TTC.

In men

We've devoted the whole of the next chapter to male-factor infertility, so we'll keep this brief:

1 **Sperm** In short, three things can be wrong with your sperm: a low sperm count (at its most extreme, this is known as azoospermia), sperm that don't move properly (low motility) and abnormally shaped sperm (two heads/tails, no heads/tails – a few of either is normal).

2 **Testicles** Infections, surgery, congenital issues, a history of cancer or undescended testicles (which goes unaddressed well into adulthood surprisingly frequently, according to our urologist podcast guest, Jonathan Ramsay) can all have an effect.

3 **Drugs** The NHS lists sulfasalazine, an anti-inflammatory used to treat Crohn's and rheumatoid arthritis, and medicines used in chemotherapy as ones which might affect sperm count and production. And the rumours about -roids are true: body-building enthusiasts should ditch anabolic steroids. Certain herbal remedies, such as root extracts of the Chinese herb *Tripterygium wilfordii* (also known as the thunder god vine), used to treat rheumatoid arthritis and psoriasis, can also affect sperm production and reduce the size of your testicles. And again, for those at the back: don't do illegal drugs, kids.

4   **Other issues** Hypogonadism is an abnormally low level
    of testosterone, which can be caused by either a tumour
    or some illegal drugs; ejaculation disorders can also
    (obviously) have an effect on fertility.

Secondary infertility – but we've done this before!

One of the most annoying things about infertility is that it can
strike at any time. And it's not only couples with no children
that experience it. Secondary infertility refers to the infertility
experienced by a couple that already has a child or children
(conceived naturally). It can be a pretty confusing time for everyone – after all, you've done this before, surely it should happen
again? But that's not always the case. In fact, one in 20 couples
experiences secondary infertility. Just like, er, primary infertility,
it can be very painful. Yes, you are lucky enough to already be
blessed with a child – but the longing to give that child a sibling,
to create a larger family, and, indeed, to shut everyone up who
keeps asking if you're going to have another, is intense. We get it.

Secondary infertility definitely comes with its own unique
baggage. Often there's quite a lot of guilt involved. Firstly,
there's the guilt that you are struggling to give your little one a
brother or sister, then there's guilt that you're not giving them
your full attention because you're obsessed with your womb,
and guilt that you somehow don't feel that your child is enough.
In almost all cases none of these are justified, but all of them
are common and completely natural. There's also the fact that
timed sex can be even trickier with a child in the house (as if it
wasn't tricky enough).

As with primary infertility, the advice is that you seek medical help after one year of trying, unless the woman is over 36, in which case you're advised to seek help sooner.

Alison Perry, host of Not Another Mummy podcast and author of OMG It's Twins, suffered from secondary infertility, after quickly conceiving her first daughter: 'I suffer from endometriosis and PCOS, but got pregnant after just three months the first time, which seemed really fast when we were expecting it to take ages,' she explains. 'Second time around it just didn't even occur to me that it might take ages, let alone five years, which was how long it took in the end.'

Having suffered from postnatal depression after her first daughter, Alison had been nervous about getting pregnant again, something that she later felt guilty about when nothing was happening. 'I had this weird mix of emotions; I knew I wanted a second baby, but I wasn't sure I was strong enough to do it again. Later down the road when things still hadn't worked I had these layers of guilt.'

Part of that turmoil was also around providing a brother or sister for her daughter. 'I had guilt around desperately wanting to give her a sibling. She used to play mums and dads and she always pretended that she had two little twin sisters. It was heartbreaking. Every time she had a birthday it was tinged with sadness because it was another year without a sibling and a bigger age gap.'

Suspecting hormonal issues as the potential cause of infertility, Alison was put on Clomid, a drug designed to kick-start your ovaries. When that didn't work, she was put on tamoxifen, which also stimulates the ovaries. With still no positive result, she was advised to move to IVF. 'It was quite a big shock. I was like, "We're going there already?!" That was actually the point where we realised just how much we wanted another child.'

After two rounds of IVF Alison now has the twin daughters that her eldest was dreaming about. 'I can safely say that I was worrying about nothing, and having a large age gap (eight years!) has so many benefits. I wish I hadn't spent all that time feeling so guilty about it.'

When is a diagnosis not a diagnosis?

... when it's unexplained infertility. This is the frustrating-as-hell diagnosis couples receive when their tests don't show any abnormalities. They aren't alone: one in four cases of infertility in the UK are officially described as 'unexplained', according to the NHS.

Fertility Network UK (FNUK) says that couples receive this diagnosis if tests show the woman is ovulating regularly and there's nothing physically wrong with her, and the man has normal sperm. There's good news: a study cited by FNUK has shown that among those diagnosed with unexplained infertility, a third will eventually conceive over seven years, and if it's secondary infertility, almost eight in ten will conceive. Another study has shown that half of all couples with this diagnosis will conceive within two years of diagnosis.

In most cases, that's where the diagnosis road ends: NICE guidelines say that if a couple diagnosed with unexplained infertility hasn't conceived after two years of trying, they should be referred for IVF. And often it works: just because the cause of your infertility can't be explained, that doesn't mean the best available treatment won't work.

Occasionally, people might end up with that diagnosis because the basic tests aren't enough: for example, FNUK lists abnormal development of follicles and ovulation; abnormal or 'trapped' eggs; luteal-phase abnormalities and anatomical abnormalities (such as failures in the mechanism in the mouth of the Fallopian tubes, which are not regularly tested for), as possible contributors. Problems with male partners, such as DNA fragmentation, which we'll cover in more detail later in this book, may also be a factor.

Unfortunately, the NHS doesn't regularly test for these factors, so you might have to venture into private medicine to look further into it. The scientific evidence for some of the investigations you may be asked to do is either thin or disputed, so it's important that you do your own independent research before paying through the nose for a test or treatment. There's a lot of snake oil in fertility treatment.

It's also worth pointing out that very occasionally, the reason behind unexplained infertility might just be that test results are borderline, or the person reading the results might not be an expert and may miss something obvious. If unexplained infertility is your diagnosis and you aren't happy, it might be worth seeking a second opinion, if only to confirm your original diagnosis.

Further testing

If your doctor hasn't found anything wrong with you, they might suggest further tests, particularly if you are under the care of a private clinic. Here's a list of other investigations that might be suggested. Some of these tests have more evidence behind them than others, so I suggest you do your research before agreeing to pay for them.

Endometrial receptivity array (ERA)

This might be suggested if you've had a few failed IVF cycles with good embryos. It's a genetic test that is thought to identify the best time to transfer an embryo. This is a relatively recent idea, so there isn't a lot of evidence for its efficacy yet, although some small studies have been promising. It's also worth pointing out that to do it your doctor will take a biopsy of your uterine lining, which isn't a particularly comfortable process.

EMMA and ALICE tests

Admittedly the best-titled of all the tests, EMMA is another way of looking at your endometrium, this time analysing the bacteria to see how much of it is healthy and how much is 'pathogenic', whereas ALICE looks for particular bacteria that might cause chronic endometritis, or swelling of the endometrium. They're both made by the same company as the ERA tests, and are often offered to women with recurrent pregnancy loss or implantation failure. They're also done in the same way as the ERA test, with a biopsy of your uterine lining. They're relatively new additions to the wonderful world of fertility tests, and therefore there isn't a lot of evidence for their efficacy, so it's worth a conversation with your doctor if he or she recommends them, plus lots of reading before you part with your cash.

APS screening

Antiphospholipid syndrome, also known as Hughes or sticky blood syndrome, is a blood clotting disorder which has been linked to recurrent pregnancy loss, late pregnancy loss, stillbirth and a range of other pregnancy complications. If you have it, you also have a higher risk of developing blood clots in the legs, arteries and brain. The good news is, it's treatable with blood thinners such as heparin or aspirin. If you've had a few pregnancy losses, your doctor might suggest you have a blood test for it. This is a pretty common test, which has plenty of evidence behind it.

Natural killer cells and immunotherapy

The screening for, and treatment of, so-called natural killer (NK) cells is part of a relatively new branch of medicine known as immunotherapy. The first thing to say is that the evidence behind this is very limited.

Natural killer cells sound like the enemy, but they're actually not: they're a type of white blood cell present in everyone's body. Without them, our immune systems wouldn't function. They're also the most common immune cells in the womb lining at the time it's most receptive to implantation, but some studies have suggested an imbalance might prevent implantation or cause recurrent pregnancy loss. A test – either a blood test or a biopsy of the endometrium – can tell you whether you have 'too many'.

Treatment for this is known as immunotherapy and, again, the evidence for it is mixed. An intravenous immunoglobulin infusion or an intralipid infusion (usually a mix of soyabean oil, egg yolk and glycerin, which is about 3,000 calories) can be fed directly into your veins, or you can be prescribed a steroid pill to take. One last time, for luck: this is a highly experimental form of medicine. Please read up on it further before agreeing to part with your cash.

Conclusion

As I mentioned at the beginning, the diagnosis road can be long, slow and infuriating, and it will require superhuman levels of patience to get through. Hopefully, this chapter has given you some idea of when and where you can speed things up a little, and how to feel like you haven't lost control entirely.

Once you have your diagnosis, it might be that you want to (or are forced to) keep trying naturally for a little longer, or it might be that you are keen to begin the next steps as soon as possible. Either way you should now have a better idea of what's going on.

5

The Swim Team

(Gabby)

As we all know, it takes two to tango. Egg must meet sperm: *let the prawn see the cocktail!* (Thanks, Paddy, wrong book, mate.*) Anyway, if a couple is experiencing infertility issues, a problem might lie with the male partner. In fact, male-factor issues are the cause of 50 per cent of all cases of infertility (kind of makes sense?). And if you look at the stats for IVF treatment in the UK, male factor (MFI) is the most common reason for undergoing fertility treatment (this makes less sense, but I'll explain later).

With this in mind, we're going to take a deep dive into sperm. *Splosh!* Yes, I went there. It's a complex beast and certainly deserves its own book but that's not what we're here for (this time) and so I will try to give you as detailed an overview as possible.

(*Paddy McGuiness, host of a terrible, but also wonderful, dating show called *Take Me Out*. This is one of his many catchphrases. If you've never seen it, I'm sure you can lose a couple of hours watching YouTube clips.)

We're going to look at what can go wrong, what can be done and what you can expect if you get a diagnosis of MFI – all with a little help from top urologist (read as: sperm doctor) Jonathan Ramsay. We'll hear Mr Gabby's experience, and we'll also hear first-hand from Daniel Langer, who went through four years of fertility treatment following an MFI diagnosis.

What you'll find in this chapter:

- Mr Gabby's MFI story.
- Early indicators of issues with sperm.
- The whack-off races.
- Semen analysis – what to expect.
- Coping with bad results.
- Lifestyle changes that can help sperm health.
- Dan's MFI story.
- Myth busting: hot baths off the menu.

Introducing Jonathan Ramsay

We'll be hearing a lot from Mr Ramsay in this chapter. As a consultant urologist, specialising in fertility, he is one of the top voices on sperm health and male infertility here in the UK. And what a voice it is: very deep, slow and considered. It commands instant respect. And he has a very posh office near Harley Street. You almost feel you should curtsey to him, but you don't because that's silly. We tried to call him Jonathan in this chapter, as we use first names through the book, but it felt weird, so he is Mr Ramsay from here on in.

My (our) story

After months of trying with zero luck, we started to think that perhaps we might have a problem. Unfortunately for Mr Gabby, our laser beam of focus landed squarely on him. As discussed in the intro, he had experienced a swelling of the testicle (or orchitis) during a bout of the mumps in his early twenties. We had always wondered whether this might have impacted his man juice.

He had also recently discovered a varicocele – an enlargement of veins in the scrotum – which at the time we were quite relieved about, following a week of fearing he had testicular cancer. But a varicocele can cause fertility issues also. Quite the cock-tail (sorry).

When we got my husband's first semen analysis results, his GP didn't offer much by way of explanation. They didn't sound good, but according to the doctor, she had 'seen worse'. Helpful. Looking for answers, I rang the Fertility Network and spoke to a lovely woman who kindly explained that we would need to have IVF – a very specific sort called intracytoplasmic sperm injection, or ICSI. A bit of a shock.

His total number of sperm was in the healthy range, but motility was 21 per cent (normal is above 32–34 per cent) and his morphology was 1 per cent (normal range is more than 4 per cent). Mr Gabby went back to his GP, who advised a second test. While we were waiting for the second test appointment to come through, I went to see my GP. I told her about his first results and she decided not to hang about – she referred us immediately to a fertility clinic.

And so we rocked up at King's Fertility, which did another

round of tests. This time he got 66 per cent motility! And 3 per cent morphology! The doctor said that he didn't think natural conception was off the table and suggested another three or four months of trying. But at the same time, he also offered us the chance to start IVF if we wanted.

Cue us sitting in his office going 'Fuck, fuck, what should we do?' Mr Gabby kicked the ball firmly into my court. I chose to kick that ball down the road and keep trying, hoping beyond hope that we would be one of 'those' couples that gets pregnant just before starting a round of IVF. And so off we went, armed with sperm-friendly lube and a renewed determination.

Having interviewed top urologist, specialising in male fertility, Jonathan Ramsay, for the podcast, I was interested to see what he would say about Mr Gabby's sperm. I kind of thought we had only one shot at fully funded IVF with the NHS, and since we had put it off, I wanted to make sure that we were in the best possible place for that to work.

Now we arrive at Mr Gabby's third and final sperm test. Mr Ramsay had suggested additional tests as well as the regular analysis – DNA fragmentation, oxidative stress (aka ROS test – more of this on page 96) and some tests looking for bacteria in his urine. These tests were all relatively good, although morphology was back down to 1 per cent. None of the bacteria was present and he had 27 million total motile sperm. DNA fragmentation was only 8 per cent – less than 15 per cent is considered 'excellent–good'. This was measured by a test called SCSA (the other test called 'Comet' has a different scale where less than 27 per cent is good).

Mr Ramsay said we should take the King's IVF round, 'because it is funded and ready to go' but that we should be optimistic about the chances of natural conception. We continued shagging and hoping. But as you know, we ended up doing the round, which worked.

Is it the jizz?

If you're trying to conceive and haven't yet been for tests, there are a few things that might give you an indication of whether sperm is the issue. None of these things are perceivable when looking at the sperm, so don't worry about doing your own investigations into the ejaculate. Unless, suggests Mr Ramsay, there is very, very little of it, in which case this may be a clue. But we're talking extremely little. Other signs are mostly to do with your medical history.

'Men must be aware of their medical history,' he says. 'They're looking for any past surgery to the testicles or groin – in particular undescended testes or hernias repaired when they were little boys or infants, or if they have ever experienced a swollen or painful testicle post-puberty. Many people are concerned if they have had mumps as a child, for example, but mumps is only relevant if it affected the testes after puberty.'

If there is something in your back catalogue of illnesses that makes you wonder about your swimmers, you can absolutely speak to your GP earlier than you perhaps might have otherwise, as Dr Katherine pointed out in Chapter 4. They should be able to refer you for tests.

The whack-off races

Whenever he likes to get a dig in, my husband says that all my good gags on the podcast are his gags. He's not lying. Well, some of them are mine and to do with my lady parts. But a *lot* of them are to do with his adventures in semen samples.

The first time he had to do a sperm sample, he had to produce it at home and get it to the hospital within the hour. Many of you will be familiar with this, I'm sure. No pressure: just get this vial of creamy secretion across town, not too hot, not too cold *and fast*. We christened it the 'whack-off races' – chortle, chortle.

Then, when he got it to the hospital, he was desperately looking for the right place to take it to and ended up panicking and handing it to the completely wrong person. Some poor unsuspecting nurse must have had the fright of her life. Needless to say, this first pot of gold went completely undiscovered and he had to do it all over again – chortle, chortle.

When he did his third and final sample, which was the only one he had to do outside the safety of his own home (well, apart from the egg collection one), he said he could hear everything from the other rooms around him and overheard a nurse come running down the stairs and straight into a room where another poor guy was busy providing his special sauce. Cue lots of shocked shouting – chortle, chortle.

In all seriousness, the guys get accused of having 'the easy bit' and in many ways, it is – but it's certainly not without its uncomfortable moments and, ahem, challenges. The world of crusty jazz mags and saucy NHS-sanctioned VHS tapes isn't really a fun one. Do you sit down on the chair, knowing what other people sitting on it do? Can you touch anything without feeling gross? Is everyone staring at you when you leave the room? It all makes for great gags, but often it is far from funny. We all get that. But we will probably continue to make jizz jokes, because it makes it all easier.

Despite all the jokes, producing a sample can be very nerve-wracking, embarrassing and sometimes actually quite hard.* There's no real getting away from it: guys can find themselves way outside their comfort zone here. But at the end of the day, needs must, and at least you're not dealing with the dildocam.

The semen analysis

Depending on what your doctor or your clinic wants to do, you will either be asked to produce a sample at home and bring it in, or to produce it in the clinic/hospital and hand it in. (You'll be given a little tub to deposit into.) Most people find it easier to do it at home, but there are occasions when they will want you as near to the lab as poss, particularly at egg-collection time. To give an example, Mr Gabby did two at home, two in clinics.

If you do it at home, as mentioned earlier, you will probably be asked to get it to the clinic within an hour and not to let it get too hot or cold.

In preparation for producing your sample the doctor will probably give you some instructions. It's important to stick to these. They could be something along the lines of:

(*This isn't a gloat but Mr Gabby found sample-producing to be a walk in the park. I'm not going to dwell on why that is, but I'm saying it to reinforce the fact that whereas some find it hard, some find it relatively easy.)

- Ejaculate a couple of days before the test, but not within 24 hours.
- Avoid alcohol, caffeine and any naughty drugs (surely this is obvious: but nicotine, weed and coke are not friends of sperm).
- Put the St John's wort, echinacea and other herbal medications down. Avoid.

What the results mean

A regular semen analysis will tell you the following:

- Semen volume: this is the amount produced and presented in the little tub.
- Total number of sperm: the number of sperm in the entire ejaculate.
- Sperm concentration: the number of sperm per unit volume (millilitre) of semen.
- Total motile sperm (or motility): number of actively moving sperm.
- Progressive motility: number of actively moving sperm swimming in straight lines or large circles (AKA the way you need them to swim).
- Sperm morphology: the number of normally formed sperm.*
- Vitality: the number of live sperm.

(*Loads of sperm have strange or imperfect shapes – we're talking two heads, two tails, big heads, small heads, and so on, as mentioned earlier. This is totally normal and nothing to worry about. But you will need to have a certain amount of normal-shaped ones to successfully fertilise an egg. Eggs are selective.)

These are the 'normal' totals – as described by the World Health Organization (WHO):

- Semen volume (ml) <1.5
- Total sperm number (million per ejaculate) <39 million
- Sperm concentration (million per ml) <15
- Motility (per cent) 40
- Progressive motility (per cent) 32
- Sperm morphology (normal per cent) 4
- Vitality (per cent) 58

Of these various results, three will carry the most sway and will be of interest to your clinic/doctor/urologist: total number of sperm, total number of motile sperm, and morphology.

Important things to note about sperm analysis

When you open your results, or get a call from the GP or clinic, it can be terrifying to get any result outside the normal range. But it is critical to stress at this point that if your results aren't great, but they aren't terrible (as in, no sperm at all or azoospermia), it might not be cause for concern at all. 'A semen analysis is only useful when it is plumb normal, or virtually no sperm at all,' says Mr Ramsay. 'Anything in the middle may not be a great indicator of fertility ... there are no other investigations in medicine which have such biological variation but which are interpreted as being so important.'

What he means is: you can have a pretty rubbish sample one

day and a great one the next. He worries that if a couple have been trying for a baby, and their first analysis is not great, they'll just think: *We have male-factor infertility, we'll never have a baby naturally.* But this isn't necessarily the case.

It's really important that a guy has more than one analysis. Things that could impact your analysis include: whether you're tired that day, whether you've been sick recently, how much sex you've had, your ability to catch it all (remember, the best swimmers are first out, so you don't want to miss that bit).

Mr Ramsay also explains that morphology can be something of a red herring. 'Let's say someone has only 2 per cent normal forms, but has something like 30 million motile sperm – that's 2 per cent of an awful lot and so could be irrelevant.' He also makes the point that morphology is judged by the human eye so there is an element of subjectivity and potential error. 'If you are going to choose one result to take most meaning from, total motile sperm is it, but you need at least two, if not three, tests to make an informed judgement.'

Additional tests

There are a few additional tests that can be done on ejaculate (and on urine) that can give clues as to a man's fertility. These aren't carried out routinely, but if you see a urologist, they might recommend you try them.

DNA fragmentation

This basically means any abnormal genetic material within the sperm that might prevent successful fertilisation or cause pregnancy loss. You can have a perfectly normal sperm analysis but have quite high sperm DNA fragmentation, which can often come to explain a couple's diagnosis of 'unexplained infertility'.

If this test is carried out, it might be reported as an index; anything lower than 15 per cent DNA fragmentation is good. Or with a different test which reports an average where less than 27 per cent is good. Lifestyle factors can play a big role in DNA fragmentation: smoking is the big one, but also diet, stress, recreational drugs, hot temperatures in the testicular area and varicocele (aka a cluster of veins in the balls – more on these in a bit).

'This test is useful to explain the unexplained: if a couple has had all the usual tests and nothing appears out of the ordinary, high DNA fragmentation might offer an explanation, and the same can be said for recurrent early miscarriage,' says Mr Ramsay. 'The reason it is not widely adopted is that the level regarded as "normal" is set very high and someone with DNA fragmentation outside the normal levels might easily go on to conceive, so it is not so good as a screening test for fertility.'

There is no traffic-light rating for DNA fragmentation tests on the Human Fertilisation and Embryology Authority (HFEA) website, but it does say that while there is some evidence of a relationship between sperm DNA damage and the outcome of fertility treatment, the evidence is conflicting and so the test results are unlikely to impact the management of any treatment.

ROS test

This is a test for oxidative stress levels in semen: sperm produce small amounts of what is known as free oxygen radicals and reactive oxygen species (ROS) and these are needed for normal function *but* they are also dangerous to sperm in high levels. Usually, the sperm environment has antioxidants that remove these bad boys and keep levels nice and even. But sometimes this tips the wrong way and these oxygen radicals cause damage to the swimmers.

Apparently 25–40 per cent of infertile men have high levels of ROS, and it is often caused by the same culprits as we discussed with DNA frag: alcohol, smoking, drugs, heat exposure, poor diet. Infections such as chlamydia or ureaplasma can also cause high levels of ROS, so a test for these may also be sensible if high ROS is detected.

The HFEA doesn't currently have any guidance on ROS testing. This would suggest that there is limited research into it. One research paper we found from 2015 said measurement of ROS has been hampered by lack of standardisation. As such, this test shouldn't be used in isolation but can be useful when building a wider picture of sperm health.

Tests for bacteria and other germs

Certain infections can cause damage to sperm health, and so a doctor or urologist might suggest getting tested for a wide range of germs. In many cases, if these germs are detected, they can be treated with antibiotics. Probiotics may also be suggested. This relates to the body's microbiome – the colony of beneficial bacteria that inhabit the gut. We're looking for a balance between the 'good' and 'bad' bacteria in the gut, and probiotics can counteract harmful bacteria. It's a bit like a panto: everything is OK provided the good bacteria outnumber the bad.

Terms you might hear

Male-factor infertility is a catchall term for anything going wrong with the sperm side of things. It could be down to any number of things: previous illnesses, blockages, genetic issues, and so on, but unlike female infertility causes, such as blocked tubes, premature ovarian failure and endometriosis, and so on, it just gets lumped under one heading: 'MFI'.

This is the reason that it is the most common cause for IVF, as mentioned in the intro, because female issues aren't counted as one reason, so individually they don't add up to as much. This is kind of indicative of the way MFI is treated across the board (in other words, barely treated at all). But below are some things they might find:

Varicocele

This is an enlargement of veins within the testicles. These are like little heat bombs, warming up parts of the testicles that should really be kept cool and so can cause problems around low sperm quality and production. They're fairly harmless in most scenarios but *can* be a cause for lower sperm quality. Getting them checked out should establish if you need treatment. 'Ideally you need to be examined and have an ultrasound,' says Mr Ramsay. 'The relevance of the varicocele is related to how big it is and therefore how much it heats the testicles. Fifteen per cent of men have a varicocele, but less than half of them are asymptomatic. Some people find that they have an ache associated with a varicocele, or they feel a bit sore after long periods of standing, but not everyone will experience that.'

When is surgery recommended? Mr Ramsay says that if it comes as part of a package, it is probably worthwhile operating. 'If we find a varicocele, poor quality sperm, absence of a pregnancy and poor high DNA fragmentation, these people need treatment. There is increasing evidence that in some men with large varicoceles, treatment makes sense – especially when there are symptoms such as dull ache.'

Azoospermia

If a man's semen analysis comes back with no sperm at all, this is known as azoospermia. Around 1 per cent of all men and 10 per cent of infertile men have this issue. There are two main kinds:

1 Obstructive azoospermia: this means there is a blockage or missing connection somewhere in the reproductive tract. Sperm is being produced, it's just not making it out.

2 Non-obstructive azoospermia: poor or no sperm production due to defects in the structure or function of the testicles.

Obstructive azoospermia can only rarely be treated with reconstructive surgery. Hormonal treatments and medications can also help if the underlying cause is low hormone production. Lifestyle changes and the avoidance of certain toxins might help; however, usually there are no treatments that will make a man produce sperm. There is also an option of surgical sperm retrieval (SSR), which involves the collection of sperm from the scrotum using a needle or scalpel. This sperm is then used as part of an IVF–ICSI treatment cycle.

As you can imagine, the treatments are entirely dependent on your individual diagnosis, so a good chat with your doctor will hopefully shed some light on your way forward.

A word on treatment of male-factor infertility

As we all know, when a couple struggles to get pregnant they are often referred to a fertility clinic. These clinics specialise in IVF. If the couple has a male-factor diagnosis, the clinic will offer IVF with ICSI. In some cases this will work and the couple will walk away with what they wanted: a baby. But in many cases, the cause of the problem in the first place does not itself get treated. And, of course, in others, it will not work, and the couple walk away convinced that the male partner is infertile and that they won't be able to conceive.

Mr Ramsay, and no doubt countless others in the profession, doesn't agree with this and would like to see more men come forward to have further examinations and treatment where necessary: 'Infertility is a big deal, it is a proper condition with proper human consequences and therefore it needs to be investigated by someone. The time for suggesting IVF or ICSI will fix it is over. These people need proper care and support, and proper information.'

In the UK, the way NHS pathways are set up, most MFI roads lead to IVF clinics. As someone who followed that path, had success and walked away happy, you could argue that this system benefited me. But I can absolutely see the points being made by

Mr Ramsay: if something is wrong with the male partner, it is right that they should be treated for the problem.

If you or your partner find yourselves in this position, you can absolutely request further tests and to see a urologist for treatment. But you might also choose the path of least resistance – the one that leads to the fertility clinic.

Coping with bad results

Dr Jack Pearson is an embryologist and fertility coach. He says: 'Unfortunately, culturally we feel the need to be the tough guys, and sperm can get caught up in that and be seen as a measure of your worth and potential as a man – and that's just not the case. Firstly, there are counsellors within fertility clinics who can talk about these results and how they make you feel. There are also support groups online set up specifically to help guys in this situation. By attending an event like that, even anonymously, and just listening, you can get some good perspective and hopefully feel that you're not alone.

'But I think, ultimately, you've got to think about it in the same way you would any other illness. We go to the GP for all sorts of reasons. Let's say we find out that we're vitamin D deficient, we just take vitamin D supplements and don't think anything of it – we don't think that we're somehow less valuable as a person. A male-factor diagnosis should be no different.'

Mr Gabby certainly didn't enjoy the news. But he was able to cope quite well with the insult to his manhood, thankfully. 'I think luckily I was never really concerned too much about the whole emasculating thing with male-factor,' he says. 'I didn't feel like less of a man. But I think it's because I'm not a particularly macho guy anyway and neither are my friends.'

For better or worse, he found humour quite a useful tool. 'I've always been someone who makes jokes about crappy things that happen to me,' he says. 'I was happy to tell anyone who would listen – almost getting there first with a laugh before they made any judgements.'

What can you do to improve sperm health?

As already covered in Chapter 2, if you google 'how to improve sperm health' you'll get a lot of answers, from the different types of food you should scoff, vitamins and supplements, and a load of lifestyle advice. If you go to a nutritionist, they will no doubt give you a diet plan of ingredients that are good for swimmers. We're going to steer away from that because, while we're sure it all helps, there isn't much evidence around it. But there are some key points that you should consider:

- Give up the fags: smoking is really bad for sperm. The warnings on the packets aren't lying. It causes oxidative stress and DNA fragmentation and should definitely be avoided if you're trying to conceive.
- Stay away from anabolic steroids and other protein-based gym supplements.
- Maintain a healthy weight: being overweight can impact fertility. Ideally, you want your BMI to be below 25.
- Cut down on booze and caffeine: excessive alcohol and caffeine consumption isn't great for your little

guys. Most experts will tell you that it's fine to have a glass of wine and cup of coffee here and there, but don't go crazy.

- Exercise: this is a complex one because the message is exercise, but not too much. Keeping fit is great for sperm health; exhausting yourself running marathons and doing spinning classes isn't.
- Keep the boys cool: if your testicles are to produce their best work, they need to avoid excessive heat. No need to wear an ice pack in your boxers, but give the saunas a swerve, wear loose boxers and, if you work in a hot environment, take regular breaks outside. If you sit at a desk all day, remember to get up and go for a walk often.
- Eat a balanced diet: if you're getting your five a day, you're laughing. If not, eat as well as you can and reduce the things that we know aren't good for us (mainly fatty, sugary foods).

Dan's MFI story

Daniel Langer is a consultant paediatrician. He was diagnosed with male-factor infertility in 2016 and, after four years of fertility treatment, he and his wife Clare welcomed baby Percy in late 2020. Here is his story: 'We got married in 2016 and had started trying a year or so before. Six months after our wedding we realised that nothing was happening, so we thought that we'd get things checked. We weren't getting any younger, and lots of our friends already had kids. We felt that age could go against us.

'We had the first initial tests via our GP, and they came back to say that my sperm count was low, motility was rubbish and morphology not much better. We were both shocked, and when I repeated the sample it was the same. The next thing we knew, just three months later, we were told that we needed IVF to have any chance at conceiving. The GP was amazing, but that was the road the fertility clinic sent us down without question.

'I'm a paediatric doctor and it had been so long since I did obstetrics and gynaecology that I really didn't know what we were walking into. I think we were quite naive at this stage. After further investigations for both of us, we applied for NHS funding and got one fresh and two frozen transfers funded on the NHS, so we thought that should be OK. You just think: *Hopefully it will just work*.

'At this point, the stigma that exists around low sperm counts didn't really hit me – I just thought: *I really want children, that's a bit rubbish – everyone else has got kids*. I wasn't worried about feeling less of a man.

'I was struck that the male side of infertility didn't seem to be dealt with. It was all about IVF. No one offered any advice or investigated thoroughly why I had a problem or what I could do to help. The whole focus is on the woman and, as a man, you end up seeing a gynaecologist because that's who works in the fertility clinic.

'We immediately started reading up ourselves to see what more we could do. We didn't have any "lifestyle factors" and we were aware of the basic stuff like, "don't wear Lycra or sit in hot tubs" but nothing more. Four IVF cycles (five embryos) and two miscarriages in, we decided to change clinic and see a fertility nutritionist. Clare had met and heard about Melanie Brown and we got diet and lifestyle plans from her and some supplements. She was the *first* person who acknowledged my infertility, spoke to and looked at me and said that I could do something about it.

'I work in a hospital, and Clare found out that a urologist with an interest in male infertility worked there, so I asked if I could have a casual chat with him; I knew he had long waiting lists, so it was a bit of a perk that I could chat to him over lunch. He had a lengthy chat with me about DNA fragmentation, varicoceles, and so on, and we ended up doing some further tests.

'It was quite embarrassing having a colleague check my balls, but I just got on with it! I should have been physically examined at our first-ever fertility appointment really. He found a varicocele and sent me to a radiologist for a closer look. They said that it was a small one, but suggested embolising it [stopping the blood flow] to see if it made a difference. I knew that it might not have been the cause of the problem, but I thought we might as well tick that box. The procedure was absolutely fine. I was more worried about who was doing it, because I work in the hospital! But it was painless and over really quickly.

'My private DNA fragmentation test came back quite high, so I followed a three-month nutrition, supplement and lifestyle plan. The repeat test came back with better results, but it's impossible to know if the plan made any real difference. DNA fragmentation is not very well standardised and so we took it all with a pinch of salt. I get the logic behind it all, but the evidence is scant.

'At the same time, Clare also had uterine surgery following a further miscarriage, and it became all about the marginal gains for us. We did two back-to-back fresh IVF cycles to bank more embryos at our new clinic. We weren't getting any younger. Family to us has always meant more than one child.

'Throughout the whole IVF process we lost eight embryos, over five embryo transfers – three of those were double transfers.

We very sadly had three miscarriages. This was all within three years, so it was very intense emotionally, mentally, physically and financially. Life became more and more on hold.

'It definitely affected me. I felt guilty. I kept thinking, *Clare's going through this because of me. If she was with someone else she could have got pregnant easily. It's all my fault!* I'm not very good at talking about my emotions and I don't often open up about these things, but there were a couple of times when I broke down crying in the car.

'I think, ultimately, that Clare helped me to realise she wanted to be with me and not anyone else – and we were in it together. We always called it "our infertility" and I've got more open with others as the years have gone on. I hate to think about how many other couples are struggling to conceive and going through the pain we have. But they are not alone.

'We finally had success last February and now have a son. I honestly couldn't tell what we did differently or if any of the changes we made had an impact. I guess it was just fundamental for us to know that we were doing everything we could possibly do, within the limits of our mental health, finances and being sensible. We know IVF is a cruel, painful and expensive lottery. It's also a mostly private industry that requires a great deal of navigation and self-advocacy, which isn't easy. But I'm so proud to say that Percy is an IVF baby!

'As a doctor, I do feel that male-factor issues need to be a more integral part of the diagnostic process. Perhaps we need more urologists specialising in male infertility to be associated with clinics. If a problem has been found with the male partner, it should be a basic right to have a full check-up and be thoroughly investigated, with advice and support given. Nutritionists should be part of the process, too. If there's a way you can improve sperm, and increase your chances of natural conception and/or IVF, that should be explored.'

MYTH BUSTING: Men should avoid hot baths

The myth Hot baths will affect men's sperm.

When I first started trying for a baby, a friend sidled up to me at a party and said, 'Have you banned Mr Gabby from hot baths yet?' I was like, 'Errr, no! But I will do!' A quick Google search suggested that it was perhaps a thing, and so I broke the news to Mr Gabby, whose single happiest moments in life are generally in a bath, with a glass of wine, so he was devastated. Was his abstinence in vain? Or was it with good reason?

The bust: true It turns out it wasn't a bad move to ban him. 'There are some research studies suggesting that frequent hot baths where the testes are exposed to high temperature can impact on the quality of sperm,' explains Professor Tim. 'As crazy as it might sound, it makes sense to avoid hot baths, especially if the man has abnormal sperm results and is taking frequent hot baths. The reason the testes hang outside the body is to keep them cooler than body temperature, so keeping them cool is important.'

Conclusion

Male-factor infertility can be a bit of a bewildering world and you can sometimes feel that no one has your back. It's clear from talking to people that there is a desire to see much more support in the system for guys with an MFI diagnosis. In an ideal world we'll start to see this happen as more stories emerge and infertility starts to get the attention it requires.

Hopefully, this chapter has helped to inform you about some of the things you'll come across on your MFI journey and given you ideas for actions you can take. Mostly, though, we hope it has made you feel less alone. There are other guys going through this, and they're probably just like you.

6

For the Lovers

(Gabby)

For couples struggling with infertility, the pain, the anxiety and the will for it to work out do not rest solely with the person with the womb. In most cases, it's something you are going through together. You both want a baby, you're both coming up with brilliant names, imagining their future and eyeing up cute kit – you're both sad when month after month you see that single lonely line on a pregnancy test. You're a team. But when it comes to seeking help, speaking to doctors and going through treatment, the focus can very much come to rest on the woman or, in the case of same-sex couples, the partner who plans to carry. On a very basic level, this isn't really surprising – for the most part the conversation is about what's going on in their body. But it is definitely the case that more could be done to include the other person.

In this chapter we'll explore the role of the male or non-carrying partner. We'll also explore how to play both roles, for those going solo. I'll be speaking directly to the 'other half' here quite a lot, but if this is you, (a) this certainly isn't the only chapter you should read (you don't get off that lightly); and (b) both parties will hopefully get something from it.

We'll look at coping mechanisms for the times when you feel overlooked, and we'll hear some of the common experiences partners have, which might make you feel less like the only person on earth getting tired of the timed sex, frustrated by your partner's hormonal outbursts or dreading trips to the jack-off room. We'll also take a look at fertility treatment as a single person.

What you'll find in this chapter:

- Becoming an emotional-support hero.
- Our husbands break their silence.
- The TTC headfuck.
- Making yourself uber useful.
- No partner? No problem.
- Same-sex partners – the sister syndrome.
- Myth busting: 'the easy bit'.

Becoming an emotional-support hero

Going through infertility and fertility treatment can become an internal battle. You're obsessed with every twitch that happens in your body and it feels as if you're always calculating and recalculating dates, days, times, amounts, and so on. Your mind is whirling. When you're the partner, this can be quite challenging. How can you possibly keep up? We speak to relationship and sex therapist Kate Moyle, to get her top tips for navigating infertility as a couple. According to Kate, communication is key: 'One thing I would advise partners is to expect unpredictability,' says Kate. 'One of the biggest curveballs is the unpredictability that comes with the hormones, which can throw everything out and, all of a sudden, you don't understand your own body. Instead of assuming how your partner is feeling, always ask and check in to see how they're feeling.'

Speak up

Unfortunately, as the partner, you might at some points feel left out and a bit like a spare part. The doctors address your partner, not you. They're talking about their body, their hormones, their diet, their ovaries, their cycle, and so on. If this bothers you, sometimes a simple request can help to bring you back in. 'You can always ask the doctors to address you both and think of you more as a partnership,' suggests Kate. 'Make it clear that you are both eager to listen and understand what will happen and what your options are.'

Regardless of how you respond to the doctors, it's important to recognise that your partner will be the focus for a while (and this will continue when you hopefully get pregnant). Remember, however, that you're allowed to have an emotional response to the situation, too. You don't always have to be the strong one. 'Sadly, the reality is that for a time, the conversation will be focusing on your partner, and that is something you need to try to make peace with and manage any negative feeling this creates for you,' says Kate. 'You don't have to do that alone – be honest about your feelings and talk to your partner if things are getting too much.'

Your shared goal is a force for good

Whatever happens along the way, try to keep your shared goal in mind. You're both on a mission to grow your family. You're in it together. Even when you have a fight, misunderstand each other or disagree on something big, it probably isn't as big as the shared goal you're moving towards. 'There may be difficult conversations and moments ahead – remind yourselves what that shared goal is as often as possible,' says Kate. 'Try not to harbour resentment or negative feelings: talk about how you're feeling. These emotions will find a way to come out regardless, so try to bring them up as part of a calm conversation rather than a screaming row in the waiting room.'

Treat yourselves and don't forget who you are

Infertility and trying to conceive can be all-consuming. It might feel like everything you do together, and each conversation, is about baby-making. It's good to make an effort to do something completely unrelated when you can. Remember the things that you used to love doing together before your lives became ruled by a fertility tracking app and constant appointments. 'Make the space to do fun things, find little treats that remind you both who you are and why you're great together,' says Kate. 'You might decide to have a fertility-free dinner together or go and see a movie. Find ways to laugh together and take your mind off things. But don't worry if something comes up that pulls you back into fertility world – an ad on TV or a throwaway line in a film. Talk about it and move on – don't let it become the elephant in the room.'

Don't be afraid to give yourselves space

Sure, you're in it together, but it doesn't mean that you can't have some moments apart to regroup and process your feelings. You might need a little break, your partner might want some alone time – that is totally cool, as long as you both communicate and don't just retreat without warning. 'The problem is, we can go into ourselves quite a lot in the process,' says Kate. 'I think it can be quite a natural instinct, especially when you're going through something like IVF. Potentially you just want to be on your own, but you're also there as a couple, so it's about learning how you can balance those needs.

'Maybe you just say, "I'm really sorry, I'm really struggling today. I'm just going to be on my own for the afternoon. It's not that I don't want to be with you. I just need to be with me." A bit of alone time doesn't need to be a red flag, and clear communication can smooth that over.'

The TTC head-fuck – she just wants your swimmers

If you're a heterosexual couple and you're trying for a baby naturally, what started off really quite lovely can turn into a bit of a nightmare after a while if things aren't going to plan. Suddenly sex isn't spontaneous, and if your partner is tracking her ovulation, she might demand sex at times you'd really rather not. After a while, you may start to feel as if she's only really in it for your sperm. This is hard. And there aren't many worse mood killers than a crazed woman brandishing an ovulation stick that she's just peed on telling you to get your kecks off and get it done. *Now.*

If this sounds familiar and you'd like to try and change the situation, there is something you can do. But firstly, understand that she is in a very strange place emotionally, and although it might seem that she's only after your swimmers (and in truth, sometimes she is) it is also coming from a place of love. She wants to start a family with you. She loves other parts of you much more than your ejaculate, we promise.

Now, have a think about what might improve your experience of the timed sex. Is there something she could do to make the mood a bit better for you? Maybe ban the phrase 'I'm ovulating' before initiating sex? Maybe try to give you advance warning? Maybe wear those nice knickers you bought her for Valentine's Day three years ago? Whatever it is, as long as the subject is approached sensitively, there's a good chance she'll take what you say on board. And if it means she can still have your sperm at the right time of the month, she'll probably be happy to do anything.

The lads' experience

Mr Emma and Mr Gabby on their experience of infertility and IVF:

Mr Emma

The early days of TTC 'When we started trying, Emma was the driving force all the way through – both trying naturally and through IVF. She's really stubborn, and she decided she wanted a baby – and that was it. Whereas I was like, "Well, if it doesn't happen tomorrow, is that such a bad thing? We could just go to the pub." It definitely stopped being fun – both her being really sad about it and the regime around sex. It was a task rather than the exciting next bit of your life.'

Taking a back seat 'From my point of view, a lot of the process was very passive. Looking back, my main take-away was that none of the medical staff acknowledged me – it was really weird. Because most of the appointments were about what would happen to Emma next, they talked to her. Even when I tried to chime in with something, they waited until I was finished, and then just continued with their conversation with her. It felt like I wasn't part of it.'

Logical not emotional 'Being a stubborn man, plus not being really acknowledged, plus not really being treated, I think all those detach you a little bit from it all. Because of that I was a lot more logical in my reaction to whatever happened; there was no real emotion involved for me a lot of the time. I think now that it was probably a defence mechanism; I was always saying, "What should we do next?", "Let's try to find a solution." But I think that the fact that I was so detached from it didn't help me engage in the ups and downs.'

My reaction to the process 'Part of me felt my role was to keep being practical about it all, but I'm not sure she really wanted me to be that person. Neither of us knew what we were doing or how to handle it. For me, it was helpful to break it all down into bite-sized pieces, especially when everything takes so long between appointments. My question was always, "Why is it going to take so long, and how can we make it happen faster?" I always wanted to do whatever we could to move it on faster. Everything seemed to take three months and I really couldn't understand why.'

Mr Gabby

The sex 'After a while, trying naturally was just more stressful than anything else. I could see that Gabby was going a bit mad about trying to time everything, which isn't exactly sexy. Also – with sex, it's like food – the concept of having a chocolate éclair when you really want a chocolate éclair is entirely different from waking up and being forced to eat one.'

Fearing for us 'I don't think I ever felt too guilty about the male-factor issue. It was completely out of my control. But there was one night I was spilling my guts to a friend at a party, and I said, "I think I've found the thing that could actually make the relationship with Gabby not work." I didn't ever actually speak to Gabby about it.'

Creating space to talk 'A natural male instinct, in my personal experience, is to try to fix things, but obviously these things, like when she was really upset, are not something that could be fixed. But I think one thing I did recognise was that she needed to get things off her chest. I could often see that the only thing on her mind was IVF/babies, and sometimes I'd be thinking: *Why are we talking about this again*, but I realised she needed to, so I gave her the space.'

Making yourself uber useful

OK so most things are happening with your partner – but that doesn't mean you can't get busy. Here are some ways you can help and keep focused on the goal:

Gabby's experience

I remember the first time we did an injection and my husband was really quite freaked out. It was Christmas, we were at my mum's house in Ireland, my period had arrived on the 25th (Merry fucking Christmas to you too, womb), so Boxing Day was the big day – we needed to start the injections to stimulate my follicles into action.

We were watching *Harry Potter and the Chamber of Secrets*, natch, trying not to think about it as the clock hands moved steadily towards 7pm (*injection time*). I think up until that point (pun intended), it hadn't seemed real. We had been talked through the whole process in the clinic, I'd Instagrammed about it and we'd smuggled IVF drugs through airport security in a freezer bag, but until we were sitting there, unwrapping the injection and picking a spot on my tummy, it hadn't really dawned on him how intense things were about to get.

I had asked him to do the injections. I wasn't necessarily scared of them, but I wasn't quite brave enough to stick them into my own flesh. It turned out that neither was he, but it had been decided that it was his job, so there was no turning back. 'It's not right to inflict pain on the person you love,' he observed quietly. But I barely felt a thing. He really wasn't happy about it, though, and he hugged me harder than he ever has before as soon as it was done.

I think it was then that he decided to become a painless-injection champion. He spent the weeks following interrogating which ones hurt more than others and why. Why did this one bleed? Was that spot of flabby tummy the best bit? Each day he built on his strategy, and by the end of it he was confident, and my tummy had barely any bruising. I think it was his way of playing his part. Sure, I was the pincushion, but he was working hard to make it as painless as possible.

Take responsibility for parts of the treatment process

This is one of our top tips for partners wanting to support someone through treatment. It is completely normal and very common for partners to feel like a bit of a spare part when the other person is (for the most part) the one having treatment. You can't take the injections for them, you can't have a go at growing womb lining for them and, sadly, you can't click your fingers and create a viable embryo, but there are things you can do. And I have no doubt they will be appreciated.

Here is a small list of suggested areas of responsibility:

Top clerking: documents and appointments When you're going through any sort of treatment, there is usually shitloads of paperwork. We had a bursting brown card folder that I had purchased from Paperchase on one of my positive proactive days. It went everywhere with us. You also have plenty of appointments. Later in the book we'll talk about this element of treatment in greater detail, but this is a point for you partners: there's a chance that if your partner is chock full of hormones and a little distracted by thoughts of a dildocam or Fallopian tubes filled with dye, she might forget the logistics, the paperwork and to feed the cat. This is where you come into your own. You've got the folder, you've planned how you're going to get to the clinic and you'd booked lunch afterwards in that nice pizza place. You are a legend.

Top clinicianing: injections As previously mentioned, we decided early on that it was Mr Gabby's job to do the injections. But this went beyond sticking them in, it also meant working out how each one is prepped (or more, remembering how the nurse told us to prep it – fear not, someone will always tell you how they work first) and getting it right. Not having to worry about that kind of thing can be a great relief. It certainly was for me.

When it comes to administering the injections, some women quite like doing them themselves. They may want to go into a room on their own and peacefully stick themselves like a Zen princess. If that is the case, that is cool. And you must let them. But it's very much down to the individual, and there are many for whom simply looking the other way while their partner does the jab, makes the daily process a lot easier. If you are taking control of injections, don't worry, it's not as hard as you imagine, and there are little tips and tricks to make it easier. You can master these.

Top chemisting: medications Some medications are really simple to use; for example, there are pre-loaded injections that just let you point and shoot. But there are others that require a bit more from you. You might need to keep it in the fridge, remember how many mls you need, mix powers, switch needles, and so on, so you might need to put your chemistry hat on and take care of this shit. One thing to remember is that even if at first these procedures sound complicated and impossible to get the hang of, they will feel like second nature after a while, so don't worry.

Top chefing: snacks Sometimes when you're feeling low, when you're bored in a waiting room or when you've just come around from a minor op, you need someone to pull a choccie bar out of their pocket and slip it into your hand. Good snacks can get you through any situation. Well, also a good cup of tea, but no one is expecting you to carry a Thermos around with you all the time (but if you could, that would be great). Different parts of the journey require different snacks. Sometimes perhaps sugar isn't a great idea, so it'll be something else. Either way – it'll bring little moments of joy to your partner if you always have a little treat on you. And you can avoid hangry waiting-room outbursts.

No partner? No problem

Every year, millions of single people decide that they want to become parents. It's a huge decision to make and one that isn't taken lightly, but there is no reason why the absence of a long-term partner should rule anyone out of becoming a mum or dad. Going it alone can often turn out to be the best decision someone has ever made. There's something hugely empowering about taking that step and giving convention the finger. If that's you, we applaud you. We hope you haven't read this chapter and thought: *Fuck, I'm gonna miss out on all of this support!* You've totally got this. But there are definitely some things you can do to help yourself.

Author and mum of two Genevieve Roberts gives her top tips on supporting yourself through treatment on a solo journey to parenthood.

Build a support network

'This was really important to me, it would be hard to go through the process (and indeed, into the next stage of parenting) without some kind of support network. The earlier you can start thinking about this and building it up, the better.

'In the first instance you might look to friends or family, but you'll also find that if you're open and share your experience online, you'll find a huge community of people there who will offer emotional support, too. I think I'm really lucky that I'm quite an open person, because I think that if you don't build a network for yourself as you're going through it, it can feel like quite an isolating experience.'

Don't feel like you're missing out

'I've only ever done this one way, that's solo, so I guess I don't have anything to compare it to, but I'm sure there are pluses and minuses for going it alone. Sure, I didn't have anyone to help with my injections, I did them myself, but I also found it easier because I wasn't putting pressure on a relationship or thinking about anyone else's feelings.'

Allow yourself to stop or slow down

'You really have to be kind to yourself. When you're single you might not have someone there to tell you to take a day off or put your feet up. I'd recommend sorting things out with your boss, so that if and when you do need that time, you can take it and won't be tempted to just charge on and pretend nothing is happening. Slowing down is much harder when you're on your own (or at least it was for me), so be good to yourself.'

Book nice things

'There are certain moments in the process when it's great to have something lovely in the diary. After my transfers, I booked to have dinner with a good friend – it was a really nice way to relax and share the experience with someone, not just go and sit on the couch and think: *I hope this works, I hope this works.* I also booked a holiday after my official test day, just in case it was bad news and I needed cheering up.'

Pick your people

'Make sure you've lined people up to be there when you need them to be; for example, when you've had an egg collection and been under general anaesthetic, you need someone to meet you at the clinic. You're lucky, because you don't just have one partner, and you can choose the best person to ask. Perhaps you want someone to make you laugh, maybe you just want the comfort of your mum – whatever it is, you can make a choice, unlike people with a partner, you have options.'

Embrace the love

'Bringing people along with you on the journey creates a different kind of family unit, in which friends and family are even more invested in your children than they would otherwise be. I guess people feel more confident stepping up because they know that there's a little more room for that extra love.'

The sister syndrome – same sex partners

Lil and Ivy always knew that they wanted to have lots of children together. They both wanted to carry and so, using the same sperm donor, they have both undergone treatment – each experiencing being the patient and the partner.

Lil went first; she got pregnant after her first transfer, but sadly lost her pregnancy. Her second transfer worked and they have a daughter, Fern. Ivy went next, and, having had several IUIs (intra-uterine inseminations – treatment that involves directly inserting sperm into a woman's womb) and five IVF embryo transfers, she is still in the process of trying.

Feeling left out

Ivy: 'I definitely felt overlooked when we were going to appointments for Lil. But, to be honest, I didn't really mind. It bothered me a lot when Lil was giving birth and I was not being included. But at the IVF stage, I kind of distanced myself from it all. I really didn't want to get involved in the biology of it all – hormones freak me out, and I'm more focused on the end goal.'

Lil: 'I remember in our very first consultation, feeling as if I was trying to start a family on my own. Ivy wasn't involved biologically, so she was just there to support me. When they were asking basic questions about IVF or IUI I thought it would be a real group discussion, but it wasn't, it was directed at me. Even the free counselling session we did, I thought it would be about us as a family unit, but it wasn't.'

Understanding strengths

Ivy: 'I think if Lil said now that I should have been more supportive, I would regret not getting more involved, but I'm going through it now, I just don't want to be reading all the info and watching the videos, I'd rather the doctor told me exactly what I need to do. Lil has done all my injections – I just don't like getting into it.'

Lil: 'Ivy is very end-goal orientated. At the time when I was doing IVF, I wasn't really too bothered that Ivy didn't get involved in the details, although I think it would have been handy for her to be more aware of the hormone rollercoaster. She hadn't done much research, so it was kind of a shock to her when I was throwing my dummy out over things. As soon as I was pregnant it was like "Great! Now we can go back to being a normal family again."'

Ivy: 'I think my support came in other ways, like cooking more and taking care of the house and giving massages. I wanted to make sure that Lil and the baby were as healthy as possible, so nutrition became really important to me.'

Lil: 'Yeah from six months before IVF, Ivy was like "here's the menu".'

Switching roles

Ivy: 'Now that I'm going through treatment, it's totally different. Because we have Fern and because of COVID, I go to appointments on my own and it's more like a chore that I have to get through rather than an exciting thing we're doing together. And even more of a chore when it's simply not working. I just want it to work now so that we can move on.'

Lil: 'Luckily, my parents were here during Ivy's first egg collection, so I was able to go along, but I wasn't there for transfers. But COVID has definitely meant that Ivy has done a lot of it on her own. We haven't really been able to keep the consistency with Ivy's experience.'

Ivy: 'Lil has actually been really good at saying, "It doesn't matter! We'll do it again. No big deal," when it hasn't worked.'

The danger of comparison

Lil: 'One thing I would definitely say to someone going through this in a similar way to us, is not to compare your journey with anyone else's, because mine and Ivy's have been so completely different. We presumed that Ivy's treatment would go similarly to mine. We were planning, "Oh well, transfer will happen then, so Ivy will be pregnant for that and then … and so on" and it really hasn't worked out that way. You do compare – we're eating the same things, Ivy is healthier than I am and we're using the same donor – what's going on?'

Ivy: 'When it worked so well for Lil, I just assumed it would be the same for me. I chose to do IUI first, because I assumed the lower success rates didn't matter for me because I don't have fertility issues, whereas Lil went straight to IVF because she just wanted to get pregnant the quickest way possible.'

The labour ward

Lil: 'It's hard to compare our experience to a heterosexual couple's experience. We only know what we've experienced. But in terms of awkwardness, the worst was definitely during my labour.'

Ivy: 'Yeah, I kept getting shunted around the theatre and told off – "No don't sit there, sit there! No, sit there!" I felt completely in the way. They kept saying, "Oh, is this auntie?"'

Lil: 'I was like, "No, that's my wife!" But, to be fair, the fertility clinic has been really good. They know who we both are and haven't called us sisters!'

MYTH BUSTING: You've got the easy bit

The myth The man's role is simple and less important.

If you're going through treatment, whether it's at the investigation stage or IUI or IVF, as the male partner you're likely to hear the phrase 'You've got the easy bit' at some point. For complete clarity, in case there is any confusion, that is referring to you having a wank. Aren't you glad I cleared that up?

The bust: false There's no 'easy bit' in fertility treatment. It's pretty hard and rubbish, and the experience of the male partner shouldn't be diminished. It's true that women generally have to go through more invasive procedures, but producing semen samples on demand in high-pressure situations isn't a walk in the park.

'I have sat with many men in the andrology department who have had difficulties actually producing the sample,' says Dr Jack Pearson. 'In that moment, you're under a huge amount of pressure. If you don't produce a sample, you can really cause issues for the process. That's incredibly psychologically challenging for a lot of men.'

To make it even harder, you're often in a situation where you feel left out. 'The focus can be on the woman; men's feelings aren't expressed or heard,' says Dr Jack. 'It's really important to acknowledge both in the couple. None of it is easy.'

Conclusion

Going through an infertility journey is one of the biggest things that can happen to a couple. For many, it is unexpected and traumatic. It wasn't on the forward-planning list after 'get married' and 'buy a house'. But even for same-sex couples, who are perhaps more emotionally prepared for the process, it can throw up unforeseen challenges. It is hard.

Everyone is different and there's no knowing how you'll react to these trying situations. What's important to know is that you're almost certainly not the first person to feel the way you do. Regardless of what's happening and how you're feeling, there are ways to help each other through it (and even if you're on your own – to help yourself). Hopefully, this chapter has given you an idea of what might be ahead, how you might feel at different points and useful ways to support your partner through it.

7

The Admin Chapter: Finding a Clinic and Funding Your Treatment

(Emma)

Once you have your diagnosis and it's clear that you will need fertility treatment, the real fun starts: you have decisions to make. Whether you are planning to hit up the NHS for some of that sweet, sweet funding, or you choose not to pass go and collect £200, and head straight for a private clinic instead, the next bit involves great research skills and yet more patience.

Your GP or gynaecologist should explain the next step, which is usually a referral for fertility treatment. Even if you're going down the NHS route, it's worth knowing that it's *your* funding, so you should be able to use the clinic you want, as long as it takes NHS patients (the HFEA website will tell you). If you're not happy with the clinic you've been referred to, speak to the clinic you'd like to approach and ask whether you can have your funding transferred – although it's also worth a conversation with your GP or gynaecologist first, to find out why you were referred to the original clinic in the first place.

This chapter will aim to cover everything you need to know to help you choose your clinic, or to just make sure that you've been referred to the right one, as well as what your options are when it comes to funding.

What you'll find in this chapter:

- Finding a clinic – what should you be looking for?
- Success rates and what they mean.
- The NHS postcode lottery.
- Private vs NHS funded.
- It all adds up: how to read a clinic's price list.
- Your funding options.
- IVF abroad.

Finding a clinic

I don't think it will come as a surprise to any of our podcast listeners, and especially not Gabby, when I say that I am not a patient woman. After a few months of TTC I had been referred for fertility tests, and I was in the middle of another 'eight to 12-week' wait for a procedure when I decided I had had enough: it was time for us to go private.

A midwife friend had told me about a celebrity fertility specialist who had got someone incredibly famous pregnant. I was pretty sure I wouldn't be able to afford A-list celeb-level treatment, but I checked out the website anyway and came away completely baffled: as far as I could tell, their approach seemed to be mainly acupuncture and supplements.* Those weren't really my bag: I wanted cold, hard drugs.

I started googling: 'fertility clinic UK', 'best fertility clinic in the UK', 'London fertility clinic reviews'. Everything I clicked on seemed totally confusing: a list of prices for procedures I had never heard of and data on success rates, which even I could see didn't make a lot of sense. Sure, one in three people got pregnant at this clinic. But what about the *women my age, with my problem and my husband?*

Meanwhile, none of them included a price for 'soothing chat with doctor who will explain everything', or what I was *really* looking for: a 'walk in and leave later that day with live baby' package. The HFEA's website didn't help much either – where were these reviews coming from?

At one point, I tried my luck with a fertility specialist just off Harley Street who wanted to charge a ludicrous amount just to see me, but he seemed vaguely legit, and I was desperate, so off the pair of us went.

His waiting room was different from the NHS one in that there was a lot more chintz and also a big plate of biscuits, which I instantly got to work on. On the other hand, we were still waiting an hour and a half. When Dr Big Dog came out, there was a sliver of what looked like raw meat on one of his Crocs. It was red, on top of his left big toe. I couldn't stop staring at it.

We went into his office and I explained our situation while

(*I later went to that clinic for acupuncture, where I met my wonderful acupuncturist, whom we have raved about on the podcast. The clinic is actually brilliant – it turned out I just couldn't understand its website.)

the sliver of meat on his shoe glistened in the light of the tasteful greige lamp on his desk.

Because I couldn't afford *anything* – not even a scan – he relented to my demands and gave me three rounds of Clomid, along with a round of norethisterone, which would bring on my period. As we left the doctor, I squeezed Mr Emma's hand and smiled. 'This is the beginning!' I said. 'We're actually going to get pregnant now!' 'Yeah,' he replied. 'Did you see that bit of meat on his shoe?'

Obviously, that Clomid didn't work. In the end, I sat out the wait and stuck with the clinic I had been referred to by the NHS, partly because PGD, the treatment I knew we would almost certainly need, is prohibitively expensive, but mainly because I couldn't make head or tail of the price lists, and I didn't really understand what we were looking for or really what questions to ask. The whole thing filled me with so much anxiety that, for the first time in my life, I decided that having patience was the best way to go.

Rest assured it hasn't happened since.

How to choose a clinic

Even just a few years on, the HFEA's website has improved immeasurably: it now has a useful tool that helps you to look at the clinic's data by treatment, age of the woman and whether the embryos were frozen (which means that they have been saved for use at a later date) or fresh (they were transferred during the same cycle the woman's eggs were collected). All that will help you to make a much more informed decision.

As I said at the start of this chapter, even if you are an NHS patient, you should have a choice of IVF clinics. It's likely you'll be referred to the closest or most appropriate, but that doesn't mean you *have* to go there; you can ask to be transferred (although the practicalities of it mean that not many people do this). If you're unsure, it's worth doing some due diligence.

Anya Sizer is the London regional organiser at Fertility Network UK and has been through numerous rounds of IVF. She says that when you're looking for a clinic, one of the most important things to remember is that 'you are in a marketplace'. The best way to find the right place is to do the legwork: 'Choose an area, choose maybe three clinics within the area, and then go and get a feel for them,' she says. Go to open evenings, speak to former patients – do anything you can to find out what it's like to be treated there.

Message boards are not always a reliable place to go for reviews. If a clinic has helped a woman get pregnant on the first go, she's likely to have a lot of good things to say about it. If it's been a long and complicated process, her review might not be so glowing. 'You've got to remember that all of them are subjective. One person's experience of exactly the same clinic and exactly the same staff can be really different from another person's.'

The other thing Anya points out is that there is no such thing as a 'perfect' clinic. 'You just go for the better of the options for you – they've all got pros and cons. They've all got staff that will have a grumpy day or a better day. There's no perfect out there. I think you can feel quite frozen trying to pick a clinic in a buyer's market.'

Here are some factors to take into account when you're choosing a clinic:

Location

Anya says that this is the key factor: 'You've got six to eight clinic visits per IVF cycle; you want it to be doable; [getting there] shouldn't add a massive strain.' Obviously, those living in cities have a lot more choice than those out in the sticks, but even if you're spoilt for choice, location should still be a factor. It's also worth taking into account where you'll be located for most of your cycle: will it be home or work? I had to hightail it to my clinic on several occasions when I started spotting mid-cycle; fortunately (and by sheer coincidence), it was ten minutes' walk from my office.

Budget

It goes without saying that some clinics are pricier than others, but that doesn't necessarily mean that you'll get a better or fancier treatment there. Some clinics offer both NHS and private treatment, and insist that all patients receive the same level of service. Some charge more because of their location, some have nicer teas and coffees in the waiting room, others have better-known doctors. Even if you can't attend an open evening in person, many are now offering video tours or online Q&A sessions with staff.

How it feels

Although my preference was that I didn't love the clinic that focused on acupuncture, rather than hard meds, other people rave about that holistic approach. As Anya says, 'Some people want that real clinical feel, because it's very comforting. Other people want much more of a homely feel. Other people want everyone in white coats so that it feels more like a hospital.' This is why visiting the clinic is important: you need to know that the way it operates is right for you.

Specialisms

I was referred by my local gynaecology department to a clinic on the opposite side of London because it was a specialist in PGD. It meant that once my embryos had been created, they were genetically tested in-house. Most other London clinics would have had to send them away, which would have added weeks on to my wait. Meanwhile, the hospital attached to it was able to do all the extra tests I needed, so all my results were easy for the clinic to access. This sort of thing is worth considering: what treatments are they able to offer in-house? Who are the senior consultants at the clinic and what are their specialisms? Is there a clinic nearby with a specialist who might be more appropriate to your diagnosis?

A note on success rates

I haven't mentioned success rates here for a reason: in the UK, all clinics report fairly similar levels of success. But it's worth remembering that the level of success they actually have varies wildly depending on the patient.

A few years ago the two of us went to see a play called *Avalanche*, a devastating one-woman show in which Maxine Peake played a woman who was desperate for a baby. During the course of rounds and rounds of IVF a clinic made incremental changes to her protocol, each time happily taking her money and promising the next one would work. Before each round she asked, 'What are the chances of getting pregnant through IVF?' 'About one in three,' the faceless doctor replied. Towards the end, she changed her question: 'What are the chances of a woman my age, with my specific problems and my history, getting pregnant?' The answer was in the low single digits.

This is not to illustrate how depressing the numbers are, but to make the point that clinics can fudge their numbers easily by picking and choosing who they include in their statistics; for example, a pregnancy rate is different from a live birth rate: clearly, the latter is more important. Similarly, we've seen some clinics show a high birth rate, but the very, very small print adds a PS: this is for women under 35.

When you speak to the clinic, make sure you know what the live birth rate is for all their patients, and, if possible, find out if it has any data for couples in your specific situation. Can they give you any information about how they have dealt with multiple pregnancy losses, for example, or male-factor infertility? What are their numbers for women over 35? The better informed you are, the more confident you'll feel in your decision.

Questions to ask a prospective clinic

Going into a new clinic can be pretty overwhelming. Here are some things to ask while you're there:

- Is there a waiting list to start treatment?
- When I'm doing treatment, how can I contact the nurses? Will I have a direct number? What hours is the line staffed for?
- Will I have a nurse assigned to me or will it be a different one each time?
- What tests will you require me to have if I start treatment

with you? (Some private clinics might ask you to repeat tests you may already have had on the NHS – the cost of this can add up.)

- Do you have data showing live birth rates for women in my circumstances? (Take into account age and diagnosis, as well as your partner's diagnosis, if it's applicable.)
- What is your policy on patients bringing children into the waiting room? (Some clinics have separate waiting rooms for people with kids. Some patients are very accepting, but bear in mind that when you are being told something is wrong and your IVF cycle isn't going to work out for a third month in a row because your lining hasn't thickened enough, having someone's toddler ricocheting off your knees while their parents smile fondly on is sub-optimal. This is a true story.)
- Are all treatments and procedures done in-house? Is anything done elsewhere?
- Tell me about how it works when you are delivering news to patients. Who calls them? What time should I expect a call?
- How much contact will I have with my doctor during my round, or will it mainly be nurses?
- What is the process for teaching me how to inject? Can someone be with me when I do my first one?
- [If you are NHS-funded] How is a 'round' of IVF defined? (This varies by CCG.)

The NHS postcode lottery

One of the worst quirks of the NHS is that the type of funded fertility treatment you can get varies wildly depending on the whims of the Clinical Commissioning Group (CCG) in your local area.

NICE guidelines recommend that anyone under the age of 40 with infertility should be offered three full rounds of IVF (that's three egg collections and transfers of any resulting embryos), although it also says IVF is 'cost-effective' until the age of 43. A 2020 report by the British Pregnancy Advisory Service (BPAS), though, showed 80 per cent of the UK's 135 commissioning groups funded fewer than that. Three funded none at all.

There's more: just 55 CCGs allowed for unlimited transfers, whereas 19 permitted only one embryo transfer per cycle. BPAS points out that this sort of policy can backfire: if people have only one chance to transfer embryos, they might choose to transfer more than one, leading to much riskier multiple pregnancies.

This is where it begins to get a little Kafkaesque. Almost half the CCGs in question also didn't offer fertility treatment to those over 40, whereas 14 offer it only to women under 35. In three areas you need to wait a year to be referred for treatment, even if the cause of your infertility is known, whereas 16 CCGs say that couples with unexplained infertility must have been trying for *three years* before they can be referred for treatment. If that pushes you over the age limit, it's game over.

BMI is another major factor: 130 CCGs specify a maximum female BMI whereas 114 specify a minimum. Thirty-two specify a maximum male BMI as well (good luck if your man is a bodybuilder; we've heard of couples being denied IVF because the male partner's workout habit pushes him over the BMI limit: he's too hench for fertility treatment).

We could go on: the rules around same-sex couples, for instance, are draconian and deeply unfair, with many CCGs requiring people to self-fund six to 12 cycles of artificial donor sperm insemination (that's a *full year*, at about £1,500 or more a pop) before they can be referred for IVF. BPAS has called the postcode lottery a 'systemic problem'.

The frustrating thing is that the only way around these rules seems to be to move house, which is neither cost-effective nor practical. Still, it's helpful to be informed about what your local CCG offers, how far you are from the border of any neighbouring CCGs, and what they offer, too. The information should be available online, or you can ask your GP to find out.

Appealing a funding decision

If funding for an NHS cycle has been denied, you can try an appeal. We'll be honest: it's only rarely successful. The only cases we know of where patients have had success are where someone had been waiting for years for IVF then had a natural pregnancy followed by a loss just before treatment started, causing the 'waiting-for-IVF' clock to be reset, and in the case of the couple we mentioned above, where the husband was a bodybuilder.

Anya says that your GP can appeal for you (although, as GP Dr Katherine from Chapter 4 points out, it takes *hours* of paperwork, so don't be surprised if they're reluctant). You can also write to the CCG directly, or you can write to your MP.

Fertility Network UK has a helpline, which can provide advice on the appeals process. Its website also has a template for a letter to your MP. There's an outside chance that they might be able to help. What is there to lose?

Screw it – should I just go private?

It goes without saying that we are very lucky in the UK to have an NHS that is free at the point of delivery. That said, the situation is complicated: just 52 per cent of first IVF cycles in England were funded by the NHS in 2018, according to figures by the HFEA, whereas only a third of the total cycles of IVF in England were on the NHS that year.

That's why, says Anya, if you're lucky enough to qualify for free treatment under the NHS, you should seize that opportunity with both hands: '[Infertility] is a medical condition and so needs to be treated by the NHS, for everyone,' she says.

There are a few reasons you might choose to pay for treatment, if you can afford it, though: it could be a timing factor (there is nothing more frustrating than being breezily told that it's going to be 'eight to 12 weeks' until a crucial test when the biological clock is ticking audibly in the background) or it might be that you'd rather opt for a clinic which offers treatments the NHS doesn't.

There are pros and cons to both sides. As anyone who has so much as set foot inside a GP's office in the UK knows, the NHS is massively overloaded, mired in bureaucracy and has world-beating waiting lists. In our experience, using an NHS clinic feels a bit like being shoved onto a conveyor belt by a careless checkout worker: there are busy waiting rooms, spartan facilities and often the staff are trying to catch up on your history while you're in the room, which can be disconcerting.

Private clinics are quicker, obviously, and might offer tests the NHS doesn't – particularly when it comes to male-factor infertility. It's worth noting that they aren't *always* as fancy or as deferential as you'd like them to be: when you are paying through the nose for treatment, you at least expect a personal butler to greet you as soon as you set foot in the door, but often the waiting rooms are just as hectic as in NHS clinics, albeit with nicer coffee machines.

And then there's the point that they are businesses, often under pressure from investors, which need to make a profit: clinics have been known to insist on tests which aren't *strictly* necessary, although the Competition and Markets Authority, the UK's competition regulator, and the Advertising Standards Authority, are beginning to crack down on this.

So-called add-on treatments are a bit of a grey area: there's no question that your NHS clinic is administering the best available treatments without the slightest hint of snake oil, because for a treatment to be approved for use on the NHS it must be rigorously tested. That means no add-ons unless it has been absolutely proven that they're effective, although at NHS clinics you might have the opportunity to join trials for some cutting-edge medicine to find out if new treatments *are* effective. Some NHS clinics will offer add-ons for an extra fee.

Some people believe an add-on was what got them pregnant, however. The NHS would never offer you a procedure such as an endometrial scratch, for example, because the research has indicated that it makes little difference to live birth rates, but we know people who swear it's what did the trick for them. Then again, we know people who swear wearing pineapple socks during their transfer was what did the trick for them – it's all a matter of judgement.

The final point to make is that most of us can't afford the extortionate cost of private treatment, and the NHS has some of the kindest, most compassionate, hardest-working staff in the world, which makes the patients who *do* qualify for funding a very, very lucky lot.

Reading a fertility clinic's price list

Once they've decided they're going to have IVF, the first thing most people do is google 'price of IVF'. Then, after they've had a glass of wine to calm down and renegotiated their mortgage, they start saving. Once they've saved the required amount, in the distance a till rings and they can then start their first cycle. Right?

Wrong. Just because a clinic says an IVF cycle costs a certain amount – £3,500, for example – doesn't mean that's how much you're going to spend. The problem is there are additional costs that often aren't factored in.

For a start, the HFEA mandates that all fertility patients – both partners, if you are using a male partner's sperm – must have virology screening for diseases such as HIV and hepatitis before the first round, which is about £250 each. An initial consultation with a scan could be around £500, so you've already spent a grand before anyone has even mentioned an egg or a sperm.

Here are some of the costs you might need to factor in to your first round of IVF, plus some rough prices (although these vary wildly between clinics):

An initial consultation: £200
An ultrasound scan during your initial consultation: £200

HFEA-mandated blood tests, female and male virology:
£250 each (£500 in total)

Hormone profiles, three separate blood tests: £400 total

Semen analysis: £150

Medication: £1,000–£2,000

Blastocyst culture (essentially growing the embryo in a
lab environment): £500

HFEA fee: £80

Headline IVF cost (which usually includes all scans and
nurses' appointments plus egg retrieval and embryo
transfer and doctor's fees): £3,500–£4,500

Any follow-up appointments or scans after your
round: £200

Freezing of any spare embryos: £700

Total: £7,430–£9,430

Funding your IVF

As you can see, IVF is prohibitively expensive – and the price list
above doesn't even include pre-implantation genetic diagnosis
(PGD), where embryos are screened for a particular chromo-
sonal disorder, or ICSI, the process where a single sperm is
selected to be injected into an egg, for example. Without those,
many patients' treatment would be pointless.

There isn't really a good way to fund your treatment. The
obvious ones are saving, which could take years – not great for
a part of medicine that is, to put it delicately, quite time sensitive – or going into mountains of debt, either by getting a credit
card or loan, remortgaging your house or borrowing off friends
or family. None of those things feel great.

Crowdfunding is another way some people do it, although that relies on having lots of friends and a *really* good sob story, or having ready access to a celebrity with a massive social media following.

There are a few other options, though, which are worth flagging:

Access Fertility

Access Fertility is a sort of finance-cum-insurance scheme which partners with clinics in the UK and Europe to provide a refund if you don't get a baby by the end of your treatment. Its packages start at about £9,000, which is a lot, but it means that you don't have to worry about the cost of IVF racking up, because you know at the end of the number of cycles you've paid for, you will get your money back if you haven't had a baby. It offers 100 per cent refund packages, multi-cycle packages and even packages for egg donation. It's worth noting, however, that drugs aren't included.

Egg sharing

This allows you to essentially 'sell' some of the eggs you get during a round in exchange for IVF services. It was originally designed as an altruistic thing, allowing women going through IVF to donate some of their eggs to other women experiencing infertility but, sadly, a lot of people use it as a way to keep costs down.

Anya points out that it should only be done after 'robust counselling', because of the sheer number of emotional pitfalls: what if the woman you donated eggs to gets pregnant and you don't? How would you feel about a child who looks like you who you may never meet? 'There's potential for things to be quite difficult,' she says.

No-baby no-fee packages

Some clinics run their own schemes, which allow you to pre-pay for a number of cycles of IVF – so called 'no baby, no fee' deals. These have been controversial, because some experts suggest that it might encourage clinics to rush treatment or overmedicate patients, increasing the risk of ovarian hyperstimulation syndrome (OHSS), but like Access Fertility, they're a good way to keep costs from spiralling out of control.

Doing IVF abroad

What could be more idyllic? You begin injections, fly out to a rented apartment somewhere sunny, have your egg retrieval, have a transfer and then fly home, ideally with a bun in the oven.

Obviously, the reality is more complicated, but because IVF in countries such as Spain, Greece and the Czech Republic is a lot cheaper, it can be a good option for those struggling to afford it.

Like anything, there are pros and cons to treatment abroad. Obviously, the holiday element is a big one for the 'pro' column, as is the cost – although make sure you factor in how much it will cost to fly out there and pay for accommodation each time. Some people travel to countries like Spain because the regulations there make it easier to find an egg donor, plus some women from South Asian backgrounds say it is easier to find a donor who matches their physical appearance.

Many of the larger clinics abroad have either 'satellite' clinics in the UK, or have arrangements with UK-based clinics, which means that you don't have to fly out to attend routine check-ups.

On the 'cons' side, it's obviously more difficult to get to the clinic, which means you might have to take more time off work than you would if you were doing it in the UK. Organising accommodation, flights, and so on, can also be pretty stressful. Some countries won't offer treatments to certain groups – single women or same-sex couples, for example – so make sure you do your research first.

It's also harder to know what you're getting into, although most clinics work according to guidelines from the ESHRE (an academic organisation that sets out guidelines on how to carry out IVF), which also vets their success data. Not all do, though, so it's important to make absolutely sure that the clinic is upholding the highest medical standards.

If the clinic you're looking at is in the EU, look out for signs that it's registered with the International Organisation for Standardisation (ISO), which ensures clinics follow all statutory and regulatory requirements.

Take time to scrutinise those stats in the brochure: are they showing live birth rates or just pregnancy rates? Which age group is this for? If possible, get independent reviews of the clinic from other patients who have flown out there.

This is by no means a comprehensive list of everything you need to take into account, but there's a list of resources at the end of this book.

Choosing to go abroad

Emma Haslam and her husband, Adam, did four rounds of IVF in the Czech Republic before conceiving their son, Albie, via donor embryo. They now run a reproductive agency, Your IVF Abroad, which helps its clients to choose a clinic and have IVF abroad.

'We were due to have treatment on the NHS, so I lost six stone to get my BMI down to under 35, but at our second appointment we were told the BMI limits for our area had now changed to 30, so could I just go away and lose another couple of stone? I was a size 14, I was slimmer and healthier than I had ever been, I had low AMH [anti-Müllerian hormone] and I was perimenopausal – so no, not really. We were devastated.

'We left that appointment thinking: *What are we going to do now?* We contacted some of the clinics in the UK and after we had handed over between £250 and £500 for consultations, the quotations we were given were very different from the prices on their websites, which left a bad taste in our mouths. We knew we were going to have to move back in with parents and put off buying a house to pay for IVF, but I didn't even know if I wanted to go with those clinics because I felt a bit duped by them.

'We started to think perhaps we should go abroad, because we knew it was cheaper. We've both done a lot of travelling, so we are both open to doing stuff like that – it didn't feel too scary. At this point, we had been given a 4 per cent chance of IVF working with our own eggs and sperm: we knew that if we found a UK clinic we gelled with, we could maybe save up and afford one round in the UK. Looking at the price in the Czech Republic, we knew we could perhaps have two or three rounds, so that is where we started searching. I was on all the forums and all over it – it felt almost like I was putting some control back where I'd lost it in other areas.

'We organised a few consultations; because they were all free, we could then compare clinics. I felt more listened to: the BMI thing wasn't an issue, things were looked at more holistically, there were no waiting lists, and when we ended up needing to use donor eggs and sperm, there were no waiting lists for those, either. I instantly felt that it was the right decision for us.

'We were also able to make it feel like a holiday. Apart from appointments, we had time to get out and go and see the sights. It's not quite the same as going on a carefree holiday, but you are still away, and it was so lovely not to have the stresses of home life and work. I was taking blood thinners; I didn't have to go into the toilets at work and inject like I was doing before we went abroad, which was really nice. Being away from home did have a good impact in terms of stress levels, and we enjoyed that time together.

'Communication was the only complication: the English was very good, but because it tends to be done via email, it's still not always written in a way that you or I might write something. Sometimes we'd have a few emails backwards and forwards just trying to clarify and understand things.

'We did four cycles in total: one was cancelled due to

a cyst. We had already booked our flights. Now I always advise people not to book their flights unless things are properly confirmed.

'In hindsight, my initial perception that it's a lot cheaper was right, but, actually, the clinics are wonderful as well. You've got to be careful, obviously, with where you go, but the standard of the personalised care, the way that you are treated and everything, was brilliant – it also just happens to be a lot cheaper.'

Conclusion

Whether you choose to go for the NHS option or you can afford private medicine or you choose to go abroad, now is the time that you need to realise that you are about to embark on hitherto-unexplored levels of admin and expense. What's important, says Anya – and what those multi-cycle packages help you to realise – is that fertility treatment is a *course of treatment*; that is, it's usually successful after a number of cycles.

If you can find a way of funding it which recognises that – whether that's a couple of cycles on the NHS or getting a celebrity to retweet your crowdfunding campaign – it will take the pressure off the need for that first cycle to go perfectly.

8

How to Have Fertility Treatment

(Emma)

'I'm not one of those people who has IVF' – we all started out thinking that. But the fact is, 2 per cent of babies born in the UK are conceived through IVF, so if you've got to the point where you're preparing for fertility treatment, you're in great company.

The first-ever IVF baby, Louise Brown, is now in her forties, but as a specialism it is still considered relatively new. The good news is that since Louise's birth the chances of conceiving through IVF have skyrocketed: in 2018, the birth rate per embryo transferred was 31 per cent for women under 35, compared with 9 per cent in 1991, according to the HFEA. That drops the older you get: it's 25 per cent for patients aged 35–37, 19 per cent for those aged 38–39 and 11 per cent for those between 40 and 42, but the odds of conceiving through IVF are improving all the time.

What IVF *isn't* is an 'easy route' to getting pregnant. We're not sure where that stereotype came from (although celebrities such as Paris Hilton who trill 'I can choose twins if I want!', as if it's the same as going into a pet shop, don't help), but it's wrong. We'll be honest: IVF is a long, slow, physically and emotionally gruelling course of treatment, which very often leads nowhere.

In this chapter we're going to be seeing a lot more of Professor Tim. We'll go through all aspects of fertility treatment, from the weirdness of sticking a needle into yourself, to the weirdness of walking around with oversized ovaries, to the weirdness of watching an embryo being put into you. Whatever course of treatment you're planning, life is about to become very, very, weird.

What you'll find in this chapter:

- The first steps: things you might be able to try before IVF.
- What to expect at your first clinic appointment.
- High days and holidays: what does an IVF cycle look like?
- IVF protocols: what are they and how do they work?
- IVF drugs: what do they do?
- What you need to know about OHSS.
- To freeze or not to freeze, that is the question.
- Embryo grading: what is your embryologist looking for?
- Transfer day.
- The weird world of add-ons.
- Cancelled cycles.
- Myth busting: two embryos are better than one.

My story

Because of Mr Emma's translocation (explained on page xvi), IVF had been on the cards for us from almost as soon as we started trying to conceive. But we had a sort of pre-consultation consultation with a woman at the clinic we were referred to very early on in the process, and she recommended against it. 'IVF is extremely tough,' she warned. 'Better to try naturally for another six months.'

I hadn't realised it was so difficult: I thought you did some injections, then something about harvesting and fertilising eggs, and then you were pregnant. It all sounded reassuringly agricultural. Like something we've been doing for *centuries*.

The first appointment at my clinic, after we had realised there wasn't another way of putting a baby in me, was when it started to sink in that this might not be the easy ride I had imagined. Firstly, it seemed as if it was going to take *months* – they had put me on a long protocol, so they wanted me to do a month on the Pill (you what?), then a few weeks of some kind of sniffy drug, then injections, then egg retrieval (*never*, I found out, 'harvesting'). The 'actually getting pregnant' bit seemed very distant indeed.

I spent the night after that first appointment looking up IVF success rates for the first time and reading blogs by other women who had been through it, who were in a similar situation to me. One had done *13* rounds. It all seemed a lot less straightforward than I had realised.

First thing was first, though: the 'injecting' bit. This was the bit I couldn't seem to get my head around: the action of intentionally plunging a needle into my own flesh felt like the most bizarre, counter-intuitive behaviour. During the day I obsessively googled instruction videos about it. At night, I dreamed about it. I genuinely didn't think I'd be able to do it, but I was also sure that *I* wanted to be the one to do it. Doing this was *my* choice, after all. *I* was the reason I couldn't get pregnant: Mr Emma might have a chromosomal disorder, but it was my crappy body that wouldn't allow his (admittedly shonky) sperm to even have a go at fertilising my eggs. The fact that we were doing this was *my fault*, and I may as well take responsibility for it.

When the drugs arrived in their discreetly labelled (because, God forbid someone discovers a married couple is trying to have a baby), chilled box, I went berserk, giving them their own shelf in the fridge, printing out a schedule where I could cross off each injection as it happened and setting a thousand alarms on my phone, because forgetting an injection was not an option.

The first injection was to take place in the evening: I decided 9.30pm was the best time to do it because I'd almost definitely be at home by then and I didn't want to take a risk by taking the drugs out of the house. We put on an episode of *Friends*, because I needed something comforting and familiar, then I watched the minute hand creep towards the big moment. When it came, I spent five minutes fiddling with the GONAL-f 'pen' to make sure I had got the dose right, then I grabbed a roll of fat, as instructed, and hovered the needle over it. Could I *really* do this?

I closed my eyes and jabbed, winced as I felt the needle pierce my skin, pressed the button, then counted to five. It *did* sting, but nowhere near as much as I had expected.

The next morning's injection was more complicated. My alarm went off early and I got up, went to get my drugs, opened various packets and then stared, bleary-eyed and bewildered, at the vial of powder and the vial of liquid, and the two needles: one small and one *massive*. Somehow, the two substances were supposed to be combined and injected into me. It was 6am and I was being asked to do advanced chemistry.

I heard a rustle behind me. 'Do you want me to do it?' croaked Mr Emma. I felt sheepish: I was supposed to be showing everyone what a strong, independent woman I was by doing all the meds myself. But I also hadn't had coffee yet, and I couldn't figure out this damn injection. 'Yes,' I mumbled.

From then on, I did the evening jab and he did the morning one. By the end I was a mess: the drugs had left me bloated and covered in bruises, my ankles were swollen from water retention and I had started to waddle when I walked. My ovaries had ballooned painfully from the size of walnuts to the size of fists as 21 follicles all crowded into a space where one would usually grow.

Work had taken a back seat during stims (the drugs used to stimulate my ovaries during an IVF cycle), because my head was a fog of hormones and anxiety as I worried about all the things that could go wrong before the egg retrieval. Would my body just randomly ovulate early? What if there was a tube delay and we missed my appointment? *What if they couldn't find any eggs?*

I have a photograph of Mr Emma preparing my trigger shot: it's late at night and super-close up. All you can see are his face and hands as he peers at the syringe to make sure he's got it right. There's a look of tenderness on his face and I can understand why: it is, after all, one of his first acts of fatherhood.

The first steps: things you might be able to try before IVF

If you're still fairly early on in the TTC process, it's likely you've read about pills that can help some people get pregnant. Online forums are full of hopeful talk of people popping them like Smarties and getting knocked up without having to resort to needles and surgery. Obviously, it's not that straightforward, but here are the things you might be able to try before full-on IVF:

Intra-uterine insemination (IUI)

Think of this as a more advanced version of the turkey-baster method. An IUI essentially delivers semen through your cervix at the time you are ovulating. It used to be very commonly used before IVF, but because it has a comparatively low success rate, it's now generally used only in certain circumstances: for same-sex couples or single women with no fertility issues who are using donor sperm, for instance, or for couples who can't have intercourse due to problems such as vaginismus or erectile dysfunction. It is considerably cheaper than IVF, though – about a fifth of the price – so it's worth asking your doctor about if you believe it might help you.

Clomifene citrate (Clomid)

Online forums love this stuff. Because it's a pill that you take for the first five days of your cycle, it seems easy and convenient – and, crucially, needle-free. Perfect. It works by blocking oestrogen production, which tricks your body into producing more FSH, thereby forcing ovulation. But there are a number of caveats: firstly, Clomid is appropriate only for women who don't ovulate – in 80 per cent of cases, that's because they have PCOS, according to Professor Tim. Secondly, ideally your clinic will monitor you, partly so that you can time your sex or IUI perfectly, and partly to avoid the risk of OHSS (ovarian hyperstimulation syndrome). Thirdly, after a certain number of cycles, the chance of pregnancy begins to decrease; NICE guidelines recommend no more than six goes. Finally, there is an increased chance of multiple pregnancies from Clomid.

It's worth pointing out that Clomid is strong stuff: they're teeny, tiny pills, but they can have a very big impact on your emotions. It induced suicidal thoughts in me. Take this as a warning: it needs to be handled with care. Usually, it is only prescribed by fertility specialists, although I've heard of a few cases where GPs have prescribed it. Either way, you should be monitored while you are taking it.

Letrozole

Professor Tim calls this the 'new kid on the block'. Letrozole is very similar to Clomid in that it induces ovulation by cheating your body into producing less oestrogen, but it's different in that it doesn't block oestrogen production altogether. One 2014 study suggested live birth rates for women with PCOS were higher with letrozole than they were with Clomid, which is surprising, considering it wasn't designed as a PCOS treatment at all: it was originally invented as a breast cancer treatment for women who were post-menopausal. Again, ideally your clinic will monitor you for at least one cycle if you are taking letrozole, and you only have a certain number of goes before it's not worth doing any more. Again, this is usually prescribed by fertility specialists.

Metformin

One of the main issues for women with PCOS is insulin resistance: although their bodies make insulin, they don't use it effectively, which leads to weight gain and lack of ovulation. Metformin is a pill (or liquid) that works by lowering your body's resistance to insulin, thereby (hopefully) helping you to ovulate. Officially, it's licensed for use in type-2 diabetes patients, but doctors increasingly use it to help women with PCOS.

Professor Tim points out that metformin can 'have some pretty nasty gastrointestinal side effects'. For some women, a more natural alternative called Inofolic, which is available online, might regulate their cycles without the side effects.

IVF, PGT and ICSI – what's the difference?

IVF is a bit of an alphabet soup: wherever you look there are acronyms. Many people might be confused to find they have been referred for forms of PGT (more on which in a second) or ICSI, depending on what they are being treated for, rather than straight IVF. Why – and what does it mean?

ICSI (intra-cytoplasmic sperm injection)

First thing's first: it's pronounced 'icksy', *not* 'eye-see-ess-eye'. Secondly, you know the traditional image of IVF? Under a microscope, a massive needle slides into view, pierces an egg and injects a single, tiny, sperm. That's actually not traditional IVF, it's ICSI, and it's used to treat male-factor infertility conditions such as a low sperm count or poor morphology.

ICSI works in exactly the same way as ordinary IVF, apart from the fertilisation part. In normal IVF, the eggs and the sperm are put together in a Petri dish and allowed to find their own ways to one another. In ICSI, the sperm with the best motility and morphology is selected then forcibly injected into the egg.

After that, you're back on track: the embryos are allowed to develop as usual.

PGT (pre-implantation genetic testing)

This process of testing cells from an embryo falls into two categories: PGS (pre-implantation genetic screening) and PGD (pre-implantation genetic diagnosis), but just to confuse things more, it's now been lumped under one acronym, then broken down into three categories:

PGT-A (previously PGS) This screens the embryo to ensure that it has the right number of chromosomes, based on the assumption that embryos with the wrong number, known as aneuploid embryos, tend not to implant, or they lead to pregnancy loss or birth defects. The science for this isn't especially promising: it's largely seen as an expensive add-on, which hasn't been proven to increase the chances of a live birth.

PGT-M and PGT-SR (both previously PGD) are used commonly by most clinics to prevent parents with a chromosomal disorder from passing on their problems to their babies. PGT-M looks for specific conditions that are controlled by one gene, such as Fragile X, cystic fibrosis or sickle-cell disease, whereas PGT-SR looks for a 'translocation' in chromosomes (my embryos were screened this way, because Mr Emma is the carrier of a Robertsonian translocation).

If you are using one of these, your embryo will be allowed to grow for five or six days, then it will be biopsied (some of the cells will be taken and sent to a lab where they will be screened) while the rest of the embryo is frozen. Some clinics have the facilities to do this in-house; others send the cells off. Either way, it might take a few weeks for the results to come back, so you'll probably do a frozen transfer cycle one or two months later.

What to expect at your first clinic appointment(s)

Your first appointment at the clinic is a big moment: a tangible step forward in your quest to bring home your baby. It goes without saying that different clinics take different approaches: some private clinics like to avoid overwhelming patients, with just a brief consultation and a scan. That's more or less what I expected at the first appointment with my NHS clinic; instead, they squeezed in a consultation, a scan, a mock transfer, bloods and a lengthy Q&A and form-filling-in session with a nurse, as well as a cheeky sperm sample, for which Mr Emma was *not* prepared.

For Gabby, her clinic brought her and the hubs in for tests separately ahead of their first consultation so that their new doctor had their vitals before he chatted to them. Gabby's first ever transvaginal scan (and first ever trip to the clinic) happened on the hottest day of the year, on the first day of her period – a fact that she was not delighted about but, actually, found to be fine. She was actually pleasantly surprised by how quick and painless the scan was, not at all like a smear test, which she was expecting. All hail dildocam.

If this is the first time you are visiting the clinic, it may be that all you should expect is an in-depth discussion with a doctor about the next steps to reaching a diagnosis, or what exactly your course of treatment will look like. But it might be more involved than that. Here are some elements that she says you might experience at your first appointment:

Consultation

Your first appointment will involve a long conversation with a doctor, who will look through your family and medical histories and steer you through the next steps in the process. It might be that they want more tests, in which case they should order those, or it may be that you are ready to proceed straight to treatment. Either way, you should finish the consultation knowing exactly what your next steps are.

Scan

This might be part of the initial consultation with your doctor: they will perform an internal scan (yes, dildocam – something to be aware of when you are getting dressed that morning) to check your uterus and ovaries.

Blood tests

The HFEA requires both partners to have full virology screening before any treatment starts to check for HIV and hepatitis B and C, as well as other conditions, depending on your medical and travel history. The rules are quite complex: once you've done them, your treatment *must* begin within three months. Your clinic might, therefore, delay this step in the process until right before treatment begins.

Semen analysis

Even if a male partner has previously been tested, there's a chance that the clinic might require another sample, so if you are in possession of a man, prepare him for this eventuality during that first consultation.

Mock embryo transfer

This doesn't seem to happen often (in an Instagram poll we did, only 6 per cent of people had it at their first appointment), but your doctor might check your cervix to ensure that they are able to get a catheter through it. It happened at my first appointment.

Consultation with a nurse

It's likely that the next steps in the process – injections and monitoring scans – will be led by nurses, so you might have a consultation with a nurse, who will talk you through the practical side of the process. This will involve conversations about your medication (how and when to get hold of it, the practicalities of storing and taking it) plus details such as how and when to contact the clinic. Now is the time to ask questions about the nuts and bolts of the process, such as 'What are the next steps?' and 'Yes, but when do I get the *baby*?'

Consent forms

Wherever you're having treatment, you'll be asked to wade through reams of consent forms. These include (but are definitely not limited to) a form about child welfare, forms consenting to receiving fertility treatment and storing your eggs, sperm or embryos, and forms allowing the clinic to disclose your information to the HFEA and other parties such as your GP. They might also ask you to consent to donating unwanted eggs, sperm or embryos to research or even other patients (this is made very clear in the form). There will be further forms to sign if you are receiving donor sperm or eggs. If you're entering into a surrogacy agreement, get ready to be mired in paperwork until any resulting baby is in its late teens.

High days and holidays: the big moments during an IVF cycle

The strange thing about IVF is that although it seems impossibly long and drawn-out, it's actually a process that involves a few radical, earth-shaking moments, with a lot of waiting in between. You'll wait for your first appointment, you'll wait for your period, you'll wait for your follicles to do their thing so that you can confirm your egg retrieval date – then you'll wait for those embryos to fertilise, grow and finally be transferred. And *then* comes the two-week wait, which we have devoted the entire next chapter to, because it lasts a geological era.

IVF can broadly be divided into two parts: before and after egg retrieval. Here's a brief guide to those big moments before egg retrieval:

Baseline scan, then more scans

This is a trip to the clinic before your meds begin to ensure that all is well in ovary town and no cysts or other gremlins have appeared. Depending on how your clinic likes to do things, you might be asked to visit every couple of days, at which point you will become obsessed with things like number of follicles and womb lining. I had three scans between the beginning of my stims and egg retrieval.

Injections begin

Whatever protocol you're on, this is inevitable: at some point you or a loved one will end up clutching a loaded syringe in one hand and a roll of your fat in the other, wondering how you found yourself here. At this point you will be grateful for your love of carbs.

The trigger shot

We'll explain more about the drugs and how they work in the next section, but a trigger shot is administered precisely 36 hours before egg collection (although some clinics might use 35- or 37-hour intervals, so don't be alarmed if your egg collection slot seems off). It triggers your ovaries to release their eggs at the exact moment you're in theatre, which is why it's important to do it on time.

Egg retrieval (and the tea and toast afterwards)

This is one of the biggest moments of your IVF cycle. Egg retrieval takes about 15 minutes and is done via a needle, which is passed through your vaginal wall and sucks out the eggs while doctors watch on an ultrasound. It's done in a proper surgical theatre. Most clinics in the UK put their patients under 'heavy sedation', which is similar to a general anaesthetic in that you're knocked out, but it means that you breathe on your own during surgery, making recovery quicker and easier.

If you are using your partner's sperm, he will be sent into a side room while you are in theatre to have what might be the most important solo session of his life. If he's worried about performance anxiety, you can ask your clinic about freezing his sperm in advance or both producing the sample together before the egg collection. Not surprisingly, the majority of men are all right on the night. As Mr Gabby once put it: 'I've been in training for this day for a very long time.'

The doctor might write the number of eggs they've retrieved on a piece of paper or they may tell you after you wake up. They'll also let you know how many were mature – that is, suitable to be fertilised. If you're using an NHS clinic, you'll be offered the legendary tea and toast at this point, too. This will be the most delicious meal you've ever had.

After egg retrieval

Once your egg collection is over, the waiting begins. Here's what happens after the clinic has collected your gametes.

Embryo culture

Although your entire cycle up until now has been focused on you and your ability to grow as many good-quality eggs as possible, suddenly everything is out of your hands. Instead, you'll wait for a series of calls from your clinic: on the first day, they'll tell you how many fertilised; on the third day, they'll tell you how many are still growing; and on the fifth day, they'll tell you how many reached the next stage, which is known as blastocyst stage. This last part doesn't always happen: clinics sometimes decide to transfer or freeze day-three embryos. If you're doing PGT, your embryos will be biopsied on day five or six (occasionally even day seven) and then frozen. You should be aware of the general plan before your egg retrieval – that plan will be updated as the day goes on.

One of the hardest parts of this bit of the IVF cycle is hearing how many of your precious eggs and embryos have failed to fertilise or develop, but you should prepare yourself for a certain level of attrition. Professor Tim says the normal fertilisation rate is about 65 per cent. 'If you start off with 15 eggs, say, then you're down to ten fertilised eggs. Then maybe half of them make it to blastocyst, so you go down to five.' This differs according to your age and the condition you're being treated for.

Embryo transfer

This is what it all comes down to: the day your clinic puts one of your embryos back into your uterus, where it will hopefully set up home for the next nine months. If your embryos have been frozen for whatever reason – if you have a high risk of ovarian hyperstimulation syndrome (OHSS), more on which later, or you are doing PGD, or you just opted for a freeze-all cycle, this could happen weeks or even months after your egg retrieval.

Pregnancy test

We will be covering the two-week wait, the pregnancy test and the ensuing emotional rollercoaster in the next chapter, so we'll stick with the facts here. About two weeks after your transfer (if you had a five- or six-day blastocyst transferred it might be a little less), your clinic will either suggest you take a home pregnancy test or ask you to come in for a blood test. Either method is absolutely fine: a home pregnancy test will give you a binary, yes-or-no answer, whereas a blood test will show *how* pregnant you are, and give an indication of whether your pregnancy is progressing normally.

IVF protocols: what on earth are they?

One of the best pieces of IVF jargon is 'protocol'. This essentially describes the course of drugs you will take during the first part of IVF treatment to stimulate your ovaries.

There are, says Professor Tim, essentially two protocols:

Long 'agonist' protocol

You may have heard a lot of talk of 'down regulation': this is where you will experience it. Under this protocol you will spend two or three weeks switching off your ovaries – essentially putting yourself into temporary menopause – using an injected or nasal spray 'agonist' drug. After two or three weeks of that drug, you will introduce a drug to stimulate your follicles (we'll go into more detail on this in the next section), while maintaining the down regulator. Finally, you'll have a trigger shot to release your eggs.

Short 'antagonist' protocol

Instead of spending a few weeks switching off your ovaries, you'll get down and dirty quickly, starting the stimulation drug on day 2 of the cycle, then adding the daily antagonist drug to switch off ovulation a few days later. When the follicles are ready, you'll then trigger.

Although most UK clinics are now veering towards short protocols, there are advantages and disadvantages to both, says Professor Tim: 'The big advantage of the short antagonist protocol is a significant reduction in OHSS,' he says. Meanwhile, 'studies suggest that on average, there is about one less egg collected with a short protocol compared to a long protocol.

'The main outcome, which obviously is important, is live birth rate. Some older studies did suggest that the live birth rate was slightly better with a long protocol compared to a short protocol. But more recent studies have suggested that any difference is very small and there's probably no statistical difference between the long and the short.'

The Pill? Surely some mistake?

There you are, ready to get on with the business of making a baby, and there your clinic is, handing you a packet of something you're more than familiar with: yes, you're going back on the contraceptive pill. Oh, the excruciating irony.

The reality is, clinics are busy places with complicated schedules and only a few slots to use – and bodies don't always play ball. Enter the Pill: the ultimate cycle-regulating device.

'It's called programming,' says Professor Tim. It works like this: you start the Pill on the first day of your period, as normal, but then often don't do the full course. Instead, you come off on a prescribed day, the first day of the withdrawal bleed becomes the first day of your cycle, you start your stims or downregulation on the day you've been asked to, and you are ready for egg collection on the exact date your clinic pencilled you in for six months ago. Happy days.

If you're really uncomfortable using it, though, you should let your clinic know. 'There's certainly no advantage in doing it,' says Professor Tim. 'Some studies have suggested a reduced success rate with Pill programming.'

The hard stuff: what you'll be taking during an IVF cycle

That's enough pussyfooting around: let's talk about the hard stuff. There are dozens and dozens of different drugs your clinic could put you on, so instead of naming names, we'll give you the general categories. The most important thing to be aware of is that although different drugs might work for different people, most have very similar success rates, so it's really a matter of preference for your clinic.

Again, these divide into before and after egg retrieval. Some jabs may come in a pre-filled 'pen', which allow you to set the dose then inject yourself relatively easily. Others are a complicated powder-and-liquid combo, which you need to mix yourself. It can be scary, but most people manage it. Either way, your clinic should explain how to use it and show you how to inject yourself. There are plenty of videos online if you're unsure.

Before egg retrieval:

Agonist or antagonist Whether you're on a long or a short proto-col, you'll take something that ensures you don't ovulate before the clinic wants you to. This can come in the form of a nasal spray or, more often, in the form of an injection.

Stims This will be either pure follicle stimulating hormone (FSH) or a mixture of FSH and luteinising hormone (LH). The main differences here are that some are 'recombinant', or synthetically made, whereas others are, ahem, 'urinary derived': yes, they are concentrated from the urine of post-menopausal women (because that's the time when those two hormones are highest). In fact, one of the most widely used stims drugs, GONAL-f, is a distant cousin of Pergonal, which was created by an Italian scientist using thousands of gallons of urine from retired nuns (with the Pope's blessing) in the 1960s.

Trigger Having switched off ovulation, you now need to switch it back on again. The trigger shot does that, mimicking the natural surge you would have if you were going through an ordinary menstrual cycle, and causing your eggs to mature in preparation for ovulation. Trigger shots can either be in the form of an agonist such as buserelin, or pure hCG – yes, the pregnancy hormone – and can, again, be recombinant or urinary derived. If you use an hCG trigger and have a transfer immediately afterwards, it's doubly important not to do a pregnancy test early: the hormones from the drug might still be lingering in your bloodstream.

After egg collection:

Luteal support Usually, the corpus luteum left behind after you ovulate would begin creating progesterone as soon as you ovulated, but because the corpus luteums have been compromised during the egg collection in IVF, they don't function properly, so it's important to take something to support your luteal phase. Usually this is progesterone, which can be administered in the form of pills or injections (intramuscular or subcutaneous), but most often it comes in the form of pessaries, which can be used either vaginally or rectally. IVF veterans know them by many names, including 'bum bullets' and 'pants destroyers' (on account of the waxy, cottage cheese-like deposits they leave in your knickers after they melt, which then causes your pants to solidify in the wash). Our lucky friend Gabby did both pessaries and injections of progesterone.

The evidence for how much progesterone to take and how long you should keep taking it for is changing all the time. Professor Tim says that if the embryo implants, by the time of a positive pregnancy test it should have sent a strong enough signal to the ovaries to make them start producing enough progesterone to support a pregnancy themselves, meaning you should be able to stop taking supplements at that point. Some women (the two of us included) would rather keep going, just to be on the safe side: most clinics say the latest you should stop is when you are 12 weeks pregnant.

Oestrogen This thickens your lining during the first half of your cycle, helping to produce a plump, juicy home for an embryo. Synthetic oestrogen usually comes in the form of tiny pills that look a lot like the contraceptive pill, but it can also come as patches, a little like nicotine patches, which you change every few days. The box might say 'hormone replacement therapy': that's because it's often used to ease the side effects of the menopause.

If you are having a fresh embryo transfer, it's unlikely that you'll be asked to supplement your oestrogen: there's usually enough hanging around from egg collection to keep your lining thick. If you are having a medicated frozen transfer, though, you might be asked to take it: by the time I had my second frozen embryo transfer, I was taking several pills a day, as well as using patches (being on that much is unusual, though).

OMG! OHSS!

The medical establishment says that there are two main risks to IVF: the first is a multiple pregnancy (more on which later), and the second is ovarian hyperstimulation syndrome, or OHSS. It is an iatrogenic disease: it is only caused by a medical intervention (in this case, ovarian stimulation); it rarely occurs naturally.

OHSS happens when your ovaries respond *too well* to stims and swell painfully. It's caused when you trigger: the act of maturing your follicles is what kick-starts symptoms, although it may not become obvious that you are suffering until several days after egg retrieval. It can be very nasty. Although no one has died of it in the UK since 2006, according to the Office for National Statistics (although the current figures only go up to 2016), IVF patients are admitted to hospital with severe OHSS symptoms in about 1 per cent of cycles. Mild or moderate OHSS is fairly common, however (symptoms include abdominal pain, a bit of bloating, nausea, an upset tummy and sore ovaries), and the symptoms will usually go away by themselves in about a week.

Professor Tim says that one of the most obvious symptoms that it's getting severe is thirst. 'If [a patient is] getting moderate or severe OHSS, then she will start to feel thirsty because she's dehydrated,' he says. Other symptoms include weeing less (because of the dehydration), a swollen tummy (because fluid is collecting), difficulty breathing (because of fluid in your chest), and, very occasionally, a blood clot in your legs or lungs, which is indicated by a swollen, tender leg or severe chest pain.

'The pre-treatment risk factors for OHSS are being a younger woman (under 35), having PCOS, having high ovarian reserve (so a high AMH or a high antral follicle count) and having had OHSS before,' says Professor Tim.

If you're in the high-risk group, your clinic might attempt to limit your chances of developing OHSS by, for example, using a short antagonist cycle and a non-hCG trigger such as buserelin, and suggesting you freeze your embryos and delay transfer. That's because while most cases of OHSS tend to resolve themselves in seven to ten days, pregnancy can make the symptoms much worse. This happened to Gabby. When she came around after collection they told her the number of eggs collected put her at risk of OHSS, so they froze all the embryos for transfer at a later date. It turns out that she didn't get any symptoms – she thinks it was her enthusiastic consumption of coconut water what did it, but that is not based on any science, so I'll ignore her.

It only takes one: why IVF isn't always a numbers game

We've all seen those posts on forums. 'We got *three million* eggs!' some happy camper will chirp. 'My doctor is *super* impressed.'

'Oh.' Someone will respond, with palpable anxiety. 'My doctor said he was pretty happy with the four we got?'

After retrieval, once everything is out of your hands, it's very easy to sit at home and obsess over the numbers. But, as any fertility doctor worth their salt will tell you, it only takes one good-quality egg to make a baby. Although numbers are important, a few high-quality eggs are much better than lots of (a clutch of?) low-grade eggs.

Because 'what is a good number of eggs?' is such a frequently asked question, it's been the subject of a lot of investigations. One of the most respected studies was by the HFEA: it looked at 400,000 patients in its database and found the chances of a live birth continued to rise until 15 eggs. After that it plateaued. 'In other words,' says Professor Tim, 'having 30 eggs isn't any better than having 15.'

It also depends on what treatment you are having: if you are having PGD, for example, you might have a higher attrition rate than if you were doing straight IVF. But it's important to remember that although a certain number of eggs will help your chances of getting pregnant, it isn't *all* that matters. Quality is more important: 'it only takes one good egg' is a cliché, but it's true. And the only way to find out what the quality of your eggs is like is to see how many fertilised, and whether the resulting embryos become a viable pregnancy.

To freeze or not to freeze, that is the question

Embryo freezing is fairly standard practice in most parts of the world these days: it started in the early 1980s, so concerns over risks to the children produced from frozen embryos have been allayed by now.

It's a strange phenomenon to wrap your head around: siblings born from the same batch of frozen embryos could be thought of as twins; they have, after all, existed on this planet for the same amount of time. In 2020 a baby girl who was born from an embryo that had been frozen in 1992 set a record: this squidgy little newborn was 27 years old. Isn't science mind-blowing?

If you produce spare embryos, are at a higher risk of OHSS or you are doing PGT, it's likely that your embryos will be frozen if they are of a good enough quality. The way they are frozen has changed in recent years: previously, they would be 'slow-frozen', with the temperature being dropped gradually over the course of an hour or so. These days, they are vitrified (frozen suddenly), which doesn't allow for damaging ice crystals to form ('to vitrify' literally means 'to convert into a glass-like state'). They're then stored at minus 196 degrees Celsius, in labelled plastic tubes inside tanks filled with liquid nitrogen.

Your clinic will only recommend that you freeze certain embryos, usually ones that have reached blastocyst stage (day five or six) and are of 'good quality' (more on which shortly).

Freezing takes its toll on embryos: about 90 per cent survive the freeze and thaw, although many lose some cells: thawing out takes a couple of hours and during that time, the embryologist might notice that some cells have died off. An embryo can lose just under 50 per cent of its cells before the embryologist declares it to be useless – before that, it can implant successfully.

During the thawing-out process, your embryologist will also look for 'signs of life'. Inside an embryo is a liquid-filled sac: if that has begun to expand, it's encouraging. It might also begin to 'hatch' out of its shell.

It's also worth pointing out that embryos aren't the same as food: once they've been thawed out, they can be refrozen if they need to be.

There's a lot of debate about whether fresh or frozen embryo transfers are more effective; some say a wait between egg collection and transfer gives your body a chance to heal, whereas others suggest that freezing and thawing an embryo can damage it. The science indicates that there isn't much in it. A study of 2,157 anovulatory women (mainly with PCOS) published by the *New England Journal of Medicine* in 2018 found the live birth rate didn't differ significantly between frozen and fresh embryos, although the group who had frozen transfers had a lower risk of OHSS. Meanwhile, a 2020 study by the *BMJ* of 460 women with regular cycles found the live birth rate was similar for both groups.

It's your choice whether or not to freeze all or transfer a fresh embryo: either way, it won't make a difference.

Embryo grading: what your embryologist is looking for

The way clinics communicate the quality of your embryo varies wildly. Whereas some will give you a complicated-sounding rating, others will simply say that the embryo is 'good quality', but what they're looking for is pretty much the same.

The first thing they look for is how even the cells look when they're dividing: research has indicated that embryos with cells that divide evenly and are pretty similarly sized and shaped stand a better chance of implanting. They also look for the number of cells being created: on the first day, it will be one cell; by the fourth day, there should be eight cells. Once it hits five days, the embryo will be a blastocyst, with too many cells to count. It'll start to look like the very beginnings of a pregnancy, with an inner cluster of cells (inner cell mass, or ICM), which will become the foetus, and an outer ring (known as a trophectoderm), which will eventually form the placenta. One encouraging sign is if the ICM has begun to 'hatch' out of the shell (called the zona pellucida): it's the cells that have escaped which will attach themselves to the uterine lining.

At this point your clinic might give your embryo a grade: a number from one to six, representing what stage of development it's at (six is fully hatched), and two letters: one to describe the trophectoderm and the other to describe the ICM. If the cells of both are regular, it'll get an AA grade – so a stage-six hatching blastocyst with beautiful, even cells will be described as 6AA. Or, if you're at my clinic, it'll be simply described as 'lovely', which isn't quite as informative, but *is* rather nice. Confusingly, there are other grading systems as well, so comparisons between clinics can be difficult.

Professor Tim points out that all this grading is reassuring, but it can be tricksy: 'When they talk about a grade it's what's called a morphological grade: the morphology of an embryo is essentially how it looks on the outside,' he says. 'The problem is that while there is a link between the morphology and the chance of implantation, it's actually not that strong a link. The main link is not the morphological quality of the embryo but the genetic quality of the embryo: the number of chromosomes in the embryo. And that's something that you can't tell by just looking at an embryo.'

Which explains why a 6AA blastocyst might not implant, but that sad little 4CD one left in the corner still might.

Transfer day: what you need to know

Transfer day feels like the culmination of all your efforts: someone is going to put an embryo into your uterus. You are *getting pregnant*. You've spent months, or even years, waiting for this moment. You're not sure what to expect, but at the very least there should be music and dancing and a parade, which is why it's incredibly disappointing that the actual process usually takes all of five minutes, during which not a single confetti cannon is discharged.

The procedure goes like this: some clinics will ask you, and whoever is with you, to change into a hospital gown, others may not; either way, you'll be asked to climb onto a bed and put your legs into stirrups while an embryologist brings your embryo in on a long, thin catheter. A speculum will be inserted into your vagina and a nurse will use a transabdominal ultrasound (the 'normal' kind, on your tummy) to watch as the embryo is gently shot through the catheter, into your uterus.

Your clinic will ask you to have a full bladder because it makes the ultrasound clearer, and the biggest mistake transfer rookies make is to drink too much water too early. If you down a gallon of water before leaving home, you're going to be in agony by the time you get to the clinic. Our tip is to take it slowly: sip a bottle of water on your way to the clinic, then have a bit more if you don't feel it's enough. Remember that your procedure could be delayed a little, and they will press down on your bladder with the ultrasound. Also, sitting in a waiting room jogging up and down because you've had too much to drink is not a great look.

Very occasionally things go wrong: one of our podcast guests' embryologists lost the embryo on the way across the room; sometimes people's cervixes aren't accessible, for whatever reason; or an embryo might get stuck in the catheter (this is easy to fix). Although it's worth being aware of these obstacles, they're very uncommon. In most cases, by the time you leave theatre you'll be legally pregnant – or, as some people like to put it, pregnant until proven otherwise (PUPO). Whatever happens next, for the next two weeks you can wander around with a smug expression on your face, sighing fondly and rubbing your belly.

Some clinics ask if you'd like to stay in position for a few minutes to rest whereas others will suggest you lie down for a longer period (although there's no evidence that this improves your chances).

The first thing most people will want to do is go to the loo, so at this point it would be remiss of us not to repeat Professor Tim's assertion that *you cannot wee out an embryo*. No matter what happens next, going to the loo isn't going to ruin your chances of the embryo implanting. You may relieve yourself with gay abandon.

Myth busting: two embryos are better than one

The myth Having two embryos put back will increase your chances of getting pregnant.

It seems like obvious maths: two embryos, two opportunities to get pregnant. But, as the data suggests, it isn't quite as simple as that.

The bust: false It sounds like the ideal situation: bung two embryos in and you have twice as many chances of getting pregnant, or you will even have twins and complete your family in one go. If IVF has one advantage, this is surely it.

Alas, no. Multiple pregnancies are cited as one of the two main risks of IVF, and, given how effective it is now (although it doesn't always feel like it), almost all clinics recommend against multiple embryo transfers except in very certain circumstances. In fact, the HFEA launched a campaign against it in 2007: since that time, the percentage of multiple births has dropped from about 24 per cent of IVF pregnancies to below 10 per cent.

First things first: transferring multiple embryos doesn't massively increase your chances of pregnancy. A 2016 study by the University of Iowa found that women under 35 had about a 46 per cent chance of live birth if they transferred a single embryo, with about a 52 per cent chance if they transferred two. That fluctuated slightly depending on the age of the prospective parent and the number of embryos they had produced, but not hugely.

Then there are the risks if you *do* get pregnant with twins: twin pregnancies are automatically categorised as high risk, because they are more likely to result in anaemia, pre-eclampsia and gestational diabetes, as well as pre-term labour. According to the NHS, six in ten sets of twins are born before 37 weeks. There's a higher chance of emergency interventions, too: according to Cochrane, people pregnant with twins planning a vaginal birth at hospital have a 30–40 per cent chance of having to have an emergency Caesarean section.

Finally, there's a 2014 study by Michigan State University that found mothers of IVF twins were five times more likely to need a C-section and ten times more likely to have a premature birth. 'Being a twin versus a singleton at birth increased the risk for all outcomes,' said Professor Barbara Luke, the study's author.

This is not designed to scare you, but to present you with the facts: on the whole, multiple embryo transfers aren't massively more successful than singletons, but a multiple pregnancy can be riskier.

The wonderful world of add-ons

Scientists are still finding new ways to increase the effectiveness of IVF, and while some are universally declared a success, others are less so. Because we'll all try *anything* to get pregnant, even relatively unproven forms of medicine, as soon as a new test or treatment is hinted at, we are all over it like flies on cow dung. This means IVF patients are essentially human guinea pigs. This is why it's good news that the HFEA has developed a traffic light system: green means that evidence suggests the treatment works well; amber means that studies have had mixed results; and red means that it doesn't look promising. We're not going to talk you through the many and varying add-ons here, because keeping up would be a full-time job, but we will explain how the traffic light system works.

Professor Joyce Harper is one of the biggest brains in British fertility: she began her career as an embryologist and was part of the team that developed PGD (now known as PGT-M and PGT-SR), she is now professor of reproductive science at the Institute for Women's Health at University College London. She also sits on the Scientific and Clinical Advances Advisory Committee, which determines which 'traffic light' to give treatments. She has three sons, all born via IVF. She says that the panel is scrupulous about what sorts of studies it looks at: 'The gold standard is a randomised control trial,' she says. The panel focuses on live birth rate, rather than pregnancy rate. 'You could do a treatment where loads of people get pregnant, but they all miscarry. So the only thing you can look at is live birth rate, but loads of studies in the past haven't done that.'

The first step is for the panel's resident statistician to perform a systemic review of new studies that have come out looking at a particular treatment. The panel then gets together and debates what its recommendation will be.

The panel had recommended an 'amber' rating on one treatment, but after two large studies came out suggesting that it made little difference to live birth rate, they changed it to red. 'We were sure, when all the statistics came together, it didn't make any difference,' she says. 'We changed it to red – we had to. We were criticised for that. People said: "But maybe patients get pregnant quicker?" But the studies weren't looking at that.' The panel will constantly review the science as new studies come out: if research indicates a treatment is actually fairly effective, they will take that into account and change the traffic light as appropriate.

It's hard to be even-headed in this situation, but it's worth checking out the HFEA if your clinic is recommending a particular course of treatment.

We'll give Joyce the last word: 'Someone said to me the other day, "Oh, but the clinic I went to says *their* data shows ..." I said, "Look, if their data shows that this procedure works, they need to publish it. They don't publish it because it's poor data, it's not robust. And if it's not robust, it's not going to get published. And if it's not publishable, we can't consider it."' Scientists, eh?

Cancelled cycles

There was a full year between my first and second embryo transfers: part of that was taken up with a wait for more testing after my first transfer didn't work, but the rest was because of cancelled transfer cycles. One month I tried a natural cycle and didn't ovulate, the next I was bleeding heavily mid-cycle; the next, my lining was too 'grainy'. It was exhausting and bewildering and, I'll be honest, I started to lose hope. I started looking into surrogacy and adoption, thinking that my uterus was just not a very hospitable place. I remember sitting in my clinic's waiting room, sobbing my eyes out, while the nurse tried to find a consultant – *any* consultant – who could say something to console me.

Your cycle can be cancelled at any point during treatment: your follicles might not respond to stims, your eggs might not fertilise, your womb lining might not thicken. I've already mentioned the mad stuff, the embryo lost on the floor of a transfer room, for example. In 2020, thousands of IVF patients discovered a cycle of treatment could be cancelled by something completely outside of their control: a global pandemic.

This is part of the agony of IVF: you don't have control over what happens to your own body, and it's utterly maddening.

There are many ways to cope if a cycle is cancelled, but my advice is that before you do anything, acknowledge that you are about to experience grief, and treat it with the gravity grief deserves. Then go out and indulge in whatever your vice is (my chosen weapon was booze) and get ready to pick yourself back up and, hopefully, start again.

Conclusion

My last word on this subject is this: fertility treatment is a frustrating, boring, emotional and painful process, but undergoing it also puts you into a group of women who are stronger and more resilient than many. Lena Dunham poked fun at 'IVF warriors' in a piece she wrote for *Harper's* magazine, but I found it hard to laugh. Women who have been through it *are* warriors: they are more courageous, more steely, more unflappable (or less flappable?) and more empathetic than their fertile counterparts. They're also way less smug – and a lot more fun at parties.

9

The Dreaded Two-Week Wait (TWW)

(Gabby)

The TWW – what is this terrifying acronym? According to official sources, the definition is the estimated period of time between a pregnancy attempt and the date when a pregnancy test can accurately indicate if it has been successful. Roughly two weeks – hence the name.

Whether your pregnancy attempt was having unprotected sex or having a team of scientists transfer sperm or an embryo to your lady parts, for most TTC-ers, the definition of the TWW is 'headfuck'. It almost feels as though the definition of infertility could in fact be 'waiting'. There certainly is plenty of it. From hours spent sitting in waiting rooms, avoiding eye contact, to waiting for a call from an embryologist, to the biggest, most all-encompassing *waiting for a baby while everyone else pops them out.*

Really, the TWW is simply one piece in the giant puzzle of infertility waiting. But it's an important one. It's rammed full of overthinking, emotional ups and downs, internalising and just plain panicking. This chapter will talk about some of the emotional challenges of the TWW and suggest some ways to deal with them.

What you'll find in this chapter:

- What happens in your head?
- Our distraction techniques.
- Early pregnancy testing: for and against.
- The IVF TWW explainer.
- How to be PUPO (pregnant until proven otherwise).
- How to deal with OTD (official test day) and afterwards.
- Myth busting: symptom spotting during the TWW following treatment.

What happens in your head?

When I was trying (and failing) naturally, I referred to this part of the month (post-ovulation, post-shagfest, pre-period) as the hope zone. Because you've done what you can – you've had plenty of sex around roughly the right time, and as far as you're concerned you could be pregnant. For me, this came with bucket-loads of hope. I'd waltz around the place, swinging from lampposts, avoiding alcohol (just in case) and telling dentists not to do an X-ray because 'I might be five hours pregnant' (true story).

Even after years of trying naturally, when it was starting to become apparent that the au naturel style of conception wasn't going to work, I'd spend a good portion of that two weeks thinking it had. I couldn't help it – there was always a chance.

Beyond the hope, there's also the detective work. *Every. Single. Twinge.* Are my boobs sore? Did I just feel implantation? And my least favourite of all: 'Is that implantation bleeding?' (Reader, it never was.) Symptom spotting ensures that you can't concentrate on anything other than your boobs, womb and whether you feel slightly sick. Work is screwed, most conversations about *anything* else are screwed, your ability to concentrate is screwed.

Mr Gabby would be trying to communicate with me before eventually asking, 'What are you thinking about, dear?' and I wouldn't know whether to tell the truth because (a) I didn't want to get his hopes up (again); and (b) I didn't want him to think I was mad. That's how this shit makes you feel: *MAD*.

When we were talking IVF TWW – the time between my embryo transfer and my OTD (official test day), which I think was actually more like 11 days – this internal scramble had the volume cranked up to max. Seeing scientists transfer our hopes and dreams into my uterus meant that I knew it was there. *I saw it with my eyes.* That made the whole thing so much more intense. It was all I could think about.

On the drive home from the clinic I freaked out because we went over speed bumps. *What if we dislodged it?!* I walked everywhere very carefully. I worried about eating anything cold in case it took the heat out of my uterus. (This included drinking smoothies but keeping the liquid in my mouth until it was warm before swallowing.) Disclaimer: these are not necessary steps. You can drink a smoothie normally and not worry about it. Although my acupuncturist did caution against eating ice cream. One moment I would be happy and confident, the next my brain would butt in and say, 'What are you doing? You're going to end up heartbroken!' And then I would stop feeling hopeful. It was so tiring – one side of my brain fighting with the other.

The symptom spotting was off the charts. Emma had experienced a bit of implantation bleeding with her successful transfer. The fact that I hadn't had any became a signal to me that it hadn't worked. I'm so annoyed that the spectre of implantation bleeding, which drove me so insane for years, was still driving me insane until the very end. One day I was working from a hotel lobby in London Bridge when I felt period twinges. I was devastated. I started shaking and crying. My working day was over. I had to go home. Sobbing.

This was pretty much the story of my TWW: hope, devastation, hope, devastation. My OTD arrived and, as you probably know, it was good news. The wait, in all senses of the word, was over.

A professional explains the TWW: Kezia Okafor

'The two-week wait is anxiety-inducing because, like anything to do with the future, there is so much uncertainty,' explains Kezia Okafor, author, fertility-mindset coach and infertility counsellor. 'We want to be able to control it, but we can't – all humans are the same. Feeling powerless and longing for a certain outcome can be really hard.'

She explains that this causes a stress response, fight or flight, which can have a huge impact on well-being and disrupt our ability to stay calm. 'It can be all-consuming. Our brain is searching for something to give it more certainty. But, instead, we get a constant guessing game.' In order to combat the stress response it's important to understand what's happening and why. 'If we're mindful of why we feel the way we feel, and why it's triggering quite a physical response, we can calm our bodies right down.

'It's important to focus on breathing at a time like this. Meditation is fantastic for some people; it's a great thing to try, even for the first time. But I'd like to stress: if it doesn't work for you, that's totally fine, too. Many people are the same and just don't get on well with meditation.'

Another way of bringing your mind into the present and to stop fretting about the future is to break the day up into manageable chunks, says Kezia. 'Try thinking, "OK, what do I need to do today? What *can* I cope with today?" If we bring the mind back to what's right in front of us, we can more easily take steps forward without feeling overwhelmed.

'There's no right or wrong response to the situation – only what's right or wrong for you. Some people throw themselves into work, others cut themselves off – whatever works for you is the right thing as long as you're mindful of how you're feeling and why you're feeling it – rather than trying to bury it in tasks.'

Distraction techniques

If you're trying for a baby naturally, it's just not practical to spend two weeks of every single month thinking only about your uterus. With that in mind, it's good to find ways to take your mind off it. Work is a pretty good distraction in itself (although you'll undoubtedly find your mind wandering in meetings). But what about at the weekend? Or the evenings? How can you stop the fretting and the constant symptom spotting?

The TWW following fertility treatment is even worse. I've heard many a strong-minded woman say that she just wants to be put to sleep for the IVF TWW and wake up when it's over and time to test. I actually think it was Emma – but she's certainly not the only one. This is not advisable, or really possible, so forget it.

What you *can* do, whatever the particulars of the TWW you're experiencing, is make a plan to keep yourself occupied. The more your brain is occupied with something else, the less it is having an internal battle and driving you mad. With that in mind, we have come up with a list of distraction techniques. Disclaimer: none of these will work. Well, maybe a little, but not entirely, so it's good to accept that from the start. But these are all nice things, so why not fill your time with them?

See your friends – all the friends

Good chats with mates really can be a tonic. Having a chat and laughing about their shit for a while will hopefully take you away from yours. It's probably easier if they know what you're going through, just so that they can be mindful of conversation topics and not be surprised by your occasional thousand-yard stare. I actually went wedding-dress shopping with a friend during my IVF TWW. Having the focus firmly on someone else was wonderful, and we had a right giggle.

Pick up the paint brush or coloured pencils

There's something really amazing about putting all your concentration into something creative. It really can zap all those intrusive thoughts about your womb and take you away to a land of colour and staying within the lines. Either grab some paints and a brush and freestyle it, or get one of those adult colouring books – honestly, if you get lost in it you'll feel really good afterwards.

Start your own Great British Bake-Off

This is another fantastic way to take your mind off things. Even if (like me) you're rubbish at baking, it's a fun thing to do, and finding nice recipes can keep you occupied before you've even started. Also – you'll have cakes! And even if you're watching your sugar intake, no one will blame you for enjoying a little treat.

Netflix and chill (in the purest of senses)

This is definitely one of those times when you can indulge in some guilt-free binge-watching, so why not pick yourself a box set and get immersed in it? No one is judging you. Try to pick something without baby plotlines. Personally, I would recommend *Schitt's Creek* (if you haven't already devoured it), you could re-watch the *O.C.* (or *Dawson's Creek* or *Gossip Girl*) or (another personal favourite of mine) watch a series of *Love Island* that you haven't seen before – from overseas if necessary. Get grafting.

Write that shit down

It might seem counter-intuitive, but spend some time writing down how you're feeling about it all. Rather than spending all the time trying not to think about it, you can designate some time for it. Write it all down, and then you can go back to distractions again. Giving your emotions the time and space they need will hopefully give you the freedom to think about other stuff.

Doing an IVF/fertility treatment TWW?

These are some extras for you:

Pack your bags and get away

There's nothing quite like the thrill of being somewhere new to take your mind off your uterus. You could plan to go on a mini holiday with your hubby (or pals) and explore a different part of the country. Sure, your mind will come back to the TWW, it would be impossible for it not to, but there will also be lots of other things going on and fun to be had (just maybe don't go skiing). Also, I was advised against going on holiday to New York during my TWW because it was a touch too far if I needed the clinic for anything, so perhaps a staycation is wise.

Werk it, werk it real good

Now, this is a bit divisive. Some people really like to throw themselves into their work during the TWW. It's certainly a distraction and takes up a lot of the day. Others would rather avoid the potential stress of work during this period. It totally depends which camp you fall into – and how stressful your job is. I can get a bit tense at work, so I wanted to stay away from it and be a Zen princess on the couch. But if you feel like work would be good for you – then go for it.

When distraction doesn't work

Mindset coach Alice Rose helps people in many different ways, including her podcast and courses in which she encourages people to think differently about their infertility-related situation. Her process encourages people not to simply run away from their negative thoughts, or to distract themselves, but to face them, and use a reframing method to take the sting out: 'We have much more power over our thoughts than we realise. It's totally possible to train our brains to reframe what we are thinking, but it takes a little bit of practice! The more you practise, like anything, the better you get at it.

'My first step for surviving the TWW (and infertility in general) is reframe. Thoughts are illusions, so when we witness, identify and observe them mindfully we can decide what to do about them, instead of being engulfed by them.

'Mindset work prep *before* you get to the two-week wait stage is therefore key so that when you're in treatment, or if you're trying to get pregnant naturally but it's taking a long time, you're really understanding how you can begin to master control over your brain and where it loves to go when you're in the midst of this incredibly challenging time. Although, if you're reading this during the TWW, it's never too late to start; for example, you can reframe the thought: *What if I get a negative test? I feel sick with anxiety – how will I cope?* with the thought: *I notice I am feeling frightened. I take every day as it comes. I am strong and I have support.*

'My second step is presence. Make a long list of things that help to ground you in the present moment. Every day, spend ten minutes in the morning checking in with yourself. You can use a little ritual with a journal and do some free writing, or try a guided meditation or just sit and look at yourself in the mirror (it sounds a bit wacky, but it can help!) and see yourself as someone to be loved, protected and looked after. What do you need today?

'Then you can go to your list of ways to stay present and pick what you want to do. If you're working all day or have other commitments, just make sure that you prioritise it and schedule it in. You can even add a little five-minute check-in to do every single hour. Sometimes we need this when we're really going off on one in the middle of a wait.

'This list can include anything from cleaning, dancing, reading, meditating, baking, decluttering . . . whatever works for you. To make your list, you can ask yourself: what makes me feel calm and happy? Then add that to your list.

'When we're clearer about *why* we're feeling certain things – not just a big list of distractions which may or may not work depending on our hormones, or how we're feeling that day, or external circumstances that we can't control, and so on – we've got a much stronger chance of beginning to master the art of waiting.'

Early pregnancy testing: for and against

Most women who go through the TWW, particularly following treatment, fall into two distinct camps: testers and non-testers. The whole concept of the TWW is based on the fact that once conception has happened a reliable test result can only really be obtained after a certain amount of time. But there are many among us who cannot wait until that exact time, and start testing early, given that a faint second line could be detected, it just might not be that strong. If you engage with the TTC community online, you'll probably be familiar with the sight of daily pregnancy tests, all dated correctly, lined up to show the progression of a second line.

There's nothing wrong with being an early tester, it's very much a personal preference; some people find that they just need to check in each day to see if there is news from the uterus. Fair.

Clinics generally advise against it, however, just because they would prefer you to test when the result is more certain. Also, if you're doing a fresh cycle of IVF and have recently had eggs collected, there could still be traces of hCG in your system from the trigger injection.

Personally, I always wanted to wait. When I was trying naturally I would wait until my period, or test only if I was late; for my IVF round, I waited until my OTD. I think it's because, as previously mentioned, I had a lot of hope – the hope zone was a nice place to be, and I wanted to hang out there for as long as possible.

I also think, particularly during my IVF TWW, that I wouldn't have handled doing a regular test very well. I think it would have broken me. But, as I say, it's totally a personal preference. Some women would rather just know. I would rather not – until it was definite – and, to be honest, even then I didn't really want to test.

The science bit

A pregnancy test measures the amount of beta hCG, or human chorionic gonadotropin (try saying that after too many pomegranate juices). It's a hormone produced by the embryo once it has implanted, at first in very small amounts, then rising to larger amounts.

Implantation generally occurs eight to nine days after conception. If you're doing IVF, it will happen three to eight days after transfer, depending on how many days old the embryo was. If you test right after a transfer or having had sex, you won't detect hCG – some days later, you might.

The real kicker with testing early if you're doing IVF is, as pointed out earlier, that the trigger injection you take before egg collection has hCG in it, so if you have a fresh transfer after your collection and you test too early, you might get a positive result even though implantation hasn't occurred. That's what we in the business call, 'a head fuck'.

Here are some voices from the two camps:

Testing early: for

'I'm a serial tester! From 8dpo (eight days past ovulation) – even sometimes from 7dpo. I guess the main reason is that I am impatient and I just want to get it over with. Also, because I usually stop myself from doing things on the TWW and I don't want to keep myself from doing them (eating/drinking certain things, having hot baths, and so on and so on) when I'm clearly not pregnant.'

'I was a pee-on-a-stick enthusiast when I was TTC by having sex, then continued when doing IVF. In my last round I tested from the day after the trigger to my OTD, as I knew it was going to be my last round (unless we get a surprise injection of cash). I love peeing in pots and testing, and I wanted to see the science behind the trigger and how long it stays in the body. I kept them in order

to see the trigger go. I know testing early doesn't change the outcome, and I kept the hope fortress up until test day even though
I knew I should have been getting faint positives by then. My
husband doesn't know about my testing crazy-lady tendencies.'

Testing early: against

'I've *never* tested early. In nine rounds of IVF, never. For me, part
of it was the control. The doctors had given me a date, and in my
head that was what was "prescribed", and that was what I should
stick to. On the other hand, and in hindsight, it was probably
because I wanted to hang on to that little glimmer of hope for as
long as possible. My IVF stats were never good, I was set up for
disappointment every time, but it didn't make me want to get it
over and done with before it had been given its fullest chance of
success. It was helpful for me to compartmentalise, it worked,
and therefore from transfer day I shifted it as far back in my head
as possible, distraction at every turn until test day, when I would
allow it to creep back into my consciousness. Don't ask me how I
did it. I can be pretty disciplined, I guess. Even moving to donor
eggs, I still had to wait, even when I knew that success was more
likely, I couldn't change what I had always done.'

'I'm a non tester. I didn't test until my period was late or until
the official test day that the clinic gave me. Getting a negative
test when it was too early can send me into a really negative
space mentally, leading to disappointment when there should
still be hope. Also, getting a negative test close to, but before,
the test day allows me to hold out hope because "maybe it's just
too soon" when I shouldn't and it actually failed. Ultimately,
I get too in my head and it backfires either way. I always

tell myself, "The day I test on won't change the outcome," so it's better to be kind to myself and wait. It's still hard to wait though.'

Do what's right for you

Kezia Okafor says: 'I would never tell someone not to do something. Personally, I wouldn't test every day because I know it would increase my anxiety, but I totally understand that, for some people, it's a way to manage their anxiety. It gives them peace of mind and something to focus on. I think if it works for you, then do it, but if you're doing it just because you've seen others do it, I would say notice how it makes you feel because it can make a stressful situation even more stressful.'

How to be PUPO

Any two-week wait can be an anxious and hope-soaked time. One of the things that makes the TWW following treatment even more anxiety-inducing is the fact that people refer to you as PUPO (pregnant until proven otherwise). They use the P word. (Brain explodes). This basically means that your clinic will advise you to act as though you are pregnant. No drinking alcohol, no smoking, no eating 'dangerous' foods such as mouldy cheese, raw fish or cured meat.

If you're like me, you'll also be embracing the PUPO-vibe for the TWW when you're trying naturally, too (without even realising there's a cool acronym for it). The boom-and-bust style of TTC that I practised was essentially acting like an angel for my

TWW, avoiding anything naughty, then getting my period and going wild on booze and mouldy cheese.

If you're doing IVF, once you've seen your precious embryo launched into your uterus, attached to all your hopes and dreams, it's very hard not to think about it being in there and what you should do to keep it safe and cosy. But there really aren't many guidelines to follow to increase chances of implantation. It's very annoying.

That said, here are some points to note.

Get out of that bed

There was a time, many moons ago, when clinics advised bed rest following a transfer, and it does seem to have a bit of logic to it. Surely, if you don't move and lie very still for two weeks, the embryo will be able to do its thing, unimpeded by your jiggling and jaggling. *No*, this is not true. Please don't spend two weeks afraid to move. You cannot dislodge an embryo by moving about. In fact, if you don't move about, you'll affect your circulation, and that's not great for an embryo. A normal amount of moving (going about your daily routine – no marathons) will get the blood flowing and keep that womb nice and inviting.

What *is* totally cool is resting up following your transfer and spending a day on the couch watching Netflix. But getting up and down and occasionally moving about is a good thing.

Avoid hot baths and saunas

This is also a pregnancy thing, but you should probably avoid extreme heat (and cold). Excessive heat can cause damage to an embryo. You should be fine as long as you don't soak in a hot bath or hot tub, or languish in a sauna. Some people also advise against hot water bottles directly on your tummy. Some also say to avoid swimming at this time. We have asked Professor Tim, and he says that the evidence is not clear on this, but that there's no harm in being cautious and avoiding it until after your test.

Eat and drink like a pregnant woman

This bit is quite annoying. Especially because you don't actually know whether it has worked. But it is advised by clinics and everyone else with skin in the game (nutritionists, dieticians, acupuncturists, and so on) to avoid the same things as pregnant women during the two-week wait. Just to recap that includes:

- Unpasteurised cheese and milk
- Mould-ripened cheeses
- Raw or undercooked meat and fish
- Cured meat
- Raw eggs
- Caffeine
- Alcohol
- Cigarettes

Try to keep a level head about symptom spotting

Now, I'm not going to tell you not to symptom spot, because I'm pretty sure that is a medical impossibility – unless you're the most incredible internal mind-controller (scientific term), in which case, congrats, you'll nail this bit. But if, like the rest of us, your brain keeps on searching for something to grab on to, don't worry, that is totally normal, but just try to remind yourself that

(a) it could be the drugs; and (b) many women get no symptoms at all at this point.

MYTH BUSTING: symptom spotting during the TWW following treatment

The myth You'll experience pregnancy-like symptoms during the TWW.

If you spend your TWW trawling through Internet forums to see if anyone had any pregnancy symptoms during their wait, you'll find all sorts of things. Some people will say that they felt sick, some will say they had sore boobs, some might even say they had an itchy bum cheek and that they were sure that was a sign (don't believe them). This will send you off into an internal spiral, constantly trying to feel *something* from your body. But will you actually feel anything?

The bust: false Professor Tim suggests that it is unlikely. 'It is natural to look for symptoms of pregnancy at this time, but in general, it is not expected after the embryo transfer.' He even says that implantation bleeding isn't really a thing. 'Sometimes there can be some blood loss, and this is often thought to be implantation bleeding, but there is actually no evidence for that sort of thing.'

If you're doing IVF, a lot of the 'symptoms' will be down to the drugs. 'Generally, any symptoms are caused by the progesterone. There is a lot going on in the woman's

> body at that time – if it is a fresh transfer, the ovaries are collapsing back down after egg retrieval and there are hormones being taken. If implantation does occur, the hCG level will start to slowly rise, but we wouldn't expect any real symptoms until after the pregnancy test.'

How to deal with OTD (official test day)

The official test day is a specific term used during the IVF/IUI process, but a lot of the following could certainly be applied if you're testing after a cycle of trying naturally. It's all about approaching a pregnancy test with some safety buffers in case it's a BFN.

As previously mentioned, I didn't want to do any testing prior to my OTD, so I had literally no idea how things were going to go as I got closer to the day (having had my transfer on April Fool's Day, that day was 12 April and I'll never forget that). As we got closer, I started to feel the need to comfort myself if the result wasn't what I wanted. I did a couple of things that actually helped quite a lot. I made a little list of things I would do if it was negative (and if it was positive). Obviously, the negative side of the list was filled with nice things and treats to make myself feel better. The other side was mainly a reminder to breathe.

Here was my BFN list word for word:

- Buy a pair of Rogue Matildas*
- Get a pedicure

(*Expensive shoes I had coveted for a long time – check them out.)

- Go for a run
- Get drunk on delicious wine
- DELICIOUS WINE
- DELICIOUS WINE

The second thing I did was make a date with one of my best friends to meet her that night if it was a BFN and get drunk. I realise this is all making me look like a raging alcoholic. I promise you I'm not, but having been so well behaved for so long, I really thought that getting drunk would help. It did bring me a lot of comfort to know that I would see my friend and be able to laugh and cry my way through the sadness.

OTD

The way your official test day will go down will depend on your clinic. Some like you to go to the clinic and do a blood test, then give you a call later that day with your result. Others (mine included) ask you to take a home pregnancy test and ring them with the result. The difference is that blood tests are considered more accurate and presumably some clinics like to be in control of the testing. Personally, I found the home test fine, albeit terrifying.

In preparation for my test day, I purchased two pregnancy tests. I went for First Response ones, which use pink dye, because apparently this is easier to read. I doubt it makes a huge difference but for the avoidance of *any* doubt, I went with this (a recommendation from Emma).

As with any pregnancy test, they recommend using your FMU (first-morning urine) because this is when your wee is most . . .

potent. And you'll get a stronger result. This meant that pretty much the second I woke up I decided to test. It was 5.19am. Following a series of unpleasant stress dreams, I was keen to get on with it. I woke my husband up, told him I was off to the bathroom, peed into a little pot and dunked the magic wand. End of story.

How to handle a positive result

It's the moment you've been waiting for. Two little lines. *OMFG!* Congratulations! Take some deep breaths and soak up the relief. Here are some things to note:

- Don't be surprised if you don't react how you imagined. Maybe you'll cry. Maybe you won't. Maybe you'll hyperventilate. Maybe you'll be strangely calm and, dare I say it, underwhelmed. However you respond is totally normal – everyone is different and your brain is dealing with a lot right now, so just go with it.
- Don't feel pressured to tell people straight away. If your friends and family know you're having treatment and you're taking a test today, they will naturally be desperate to know the result. Don't feel you need to rush straight to tell them, but keep it to yourself (and partner) for a while if you want to. But, obviously, if you want to tell them – do! Even at 5.19am!
- Today is the day to indulge in all the baby-related googling that you've potentially avoided for a long time. Look up names, look at baby grows, search for

the trendiest changing bags money can buy – whatever it is, finally indulging is a nice feeling.

- Know that you might start to feel anxious – it's normal. Getting a positive test isn't the end of anxiety, sadly, which can generally come along and tap you on the shoulder pretty quickly, but try to focus on your result. Today, you are pregnant.

How to handle a negative result

Hello, Emma here: sneaking in to tell you about coping with a negative result. The truth is, I didn't do it well, as you will see from my story in Chapter 12 on grief. But here's what I've learned you should do:

- Recognise what you're going through. That overwhelming emotion welling up inside you is called grief, and it's awful. It's going to wash over you like waves, and its intensity might take you by surprise, but it will subside eventually. I promise.
- Book a few days off work. If you're anything like me, you're going to be a hot mess. Don't try to keep it together for your boss. There's no point.
- Share. The most healing thing I did after my negative test was my first-ever infertility-related post on Instagram. It was a picture of a little cardigan I had made right back when we first started TTC, and in the caption I confessed that we had been going through IVF and had had a negative result. The kindness that came flooding back to me got me through the next

few days: people sent me flowers and chocolates, I heard from school friends I barely remembered, who told me that they'd been through similar stuff. It was incredible. I'm not saying that you need to tell the world about it, but if you can find a friend or family member to share with, you might be surprised at the empathy you get in return.

- Find your coping strategy. Some people are wallowers: they need to spend time with their grief and slowly figure out what's next. I am a doer: I need to know what the next step is immediately, or I will go insane. Because of that, I contacted my clinic immediately. They told me someone would get back to me in five working days. Sometimes even doers are thwarted ...

Post-treatment WTF appointment

The first meeting with your clinic after a round of treatment has failed is often lovingly referred to as the 'WTF appointment'. As in, what the fuck, doctor? It's a meeting during which the clinician will hopefully give you any insight they have into why it might not have worked, and some recommended next steps.

At some point you or your partner will almost certainly mouth, 'WTF?' to each other, if not stand on the desk and scream it directly into the face of the doctor. Either way, this meeting is an important one to have.

It's fair to say, the doctors can't always give you any insight into why it didn't work – so try not to get your hopes up that they can and will tell you why you're in this position. Science is amazing, but sometimes they just don't know. The doctor will hopefully advise you on some sensible next steps and you can go home, eat a mountain of chocolate, drown in wine and probably start planning immediately for the next attempt. It's the 'determined zone' on steroids.

Conclusion

The two-week wait is one of the best, but also the worst, parts of the TTC journey. It's a time filled with hope and excitement for the future and what might be, but it also kidnaps your brain and takes it on a magical mystery tour of constant symptom spotting and internal battles about the outcome. There are definitely ways to cope with it, and you've read about a few of those here in this chapter. Take each day as it comes, and it really does what it says on the tin: after two weeks (perhaps sooner), it will be over and you can have your brain back.

10

Surviving the Daily Grind

(Gabby)

When you're struggling to conceive, it's hard to think about anything else. This is inconvenient at the weekend when your best friend asks you which pair of shoes she should buy and you're just thinking about your womb. It's much worse when you're in an important meeting and your mind keeps wandering off to think about whether you feel a bit sick or when your ovulation day is that month. Yes, work and a TTC struggle are not comfortable bedfellows. Try as you might, it's impossible to leave your emotions at the door when you go to work, so how do you cope when you're having a bad day? If you find you need IVF, how do you approach the subject with your employers? What are the rules and regulations? This chapter will explore these questions and more.

What you'll find in this chapter:

- Tips on coping with infertility stress at work.
- The career conundrum explored.
- What are your rights in the workplace? Fertility policies in the workplace (or the lack thereof).

- Telling your boss.
- Interview: TTC at the top of your game.

Werk, werk, werk

Trying to hide tears while sitting at a desk is really hard. Your computer screen is never quite big enough. Big drops of salty water rolling down your cheeks, once brushed away, keep rolling down your hand, then down your pen before dramatically landing on your notepad, creating a splashing ink pattern – like your own personal Rorschach test – inevitably giving you away to a colleague.

Alternatively, if you don't get caught in your seat, you'll try to make a break for the ladies' loos. Weaving your way through the office, head down, avoiding eye contact and trying to hide your blotchy face before bursting through the toilet door and slamming straight into your boss. *Bam!* Caught.

I became such a regular toilet crier during my TTC years that I would keep a secret make-up bag in the loo with foundation so that I could cover up my red face during emergencies. Whenever I'd get my period, or start to feel like I was about to, my day would end up derailed – in the loo, trying to cover the damage.

In many ways, work can be a really good distraction from infertility. It gives your brain something else to be distracted by – a way to keep yourself busy. This can be great. But every once in a while, particularly when you've had a negative test or your period starts, you can have a really awful day. A day when you feel very exposed and all you want to do is hide, cry and eat chocolate.

Here are some tips on surviving the stress of infertility at work:

Tell a work buddy

Telling your boss is one thing, and we'll deal with that in a moment. But if you don't feel you can do that yet (or at all), consider finding a sympathetic ear in your team: someone who you can offload your woes to on the walk to Pret at lunch, or you can send IMs to across the room if you're having a moment.

WFH if feeling wobbly

This won't work every time, but on the occasion that you're feeling a bit wobbly – perhaps you got your period or news that someone is pregnant – consider asking to work from home that day. At least if you're in the safety of your own house, you can shed the odd tear but get on with your work as best you can without the added stress of being seen.

Listen to a podcast

If your mind won't let you concentrate on work and keeps taking you back to infertility, try to break the circuit with a podcast or some music. If you can pull your mind away for long enough to calm down and feel a bit better, hopefully you can go back to your next task feeling a bit more robust.

Don't fight it

If you can feel a meltdown brewing, sometimes you're better off getting it out rather than trying to squash it down. Take yourself for a walk, have a little cry, make a call to a friend, whatever you need to do to get it off your chest, and go back with your head held high.

Avoid baby showers

For the most part, work is a baby-free zone. You've only got to worry about pregnancy announcements, baby showers and those awkward visits that people make to show off their babies when they're on mat leave. Don't feel you have to show up to baby showers or meet and greets – look after your heart, make an excuse, get out of there. You can buy your own cupcake on the way home.

The career conundrum

The woes of working mums, career breaks because of children and the difficulties balancing parenting with the job you love are quite well documented. But what many of us don't expect (and it doesn't get any airtime) is the impact that *trying* to become a mum can have on your career. On the one hand, perhaps you are ambitious and keen to progress in your chosen profession. On the other, you want to do everything you can to help your baby-making efforts. Sometimes these two things are at odds. Especially when a fertility struggle goes on for a long time.

There are no right or wrong answers here. The truth is that you have to do what is right for you. I know, that's a total cop-out. But if you honestly feel your job is getting in the way of you getting pregnant, or the stress of managing a team and a round of treatment is really doing damage to your mental health, then perhaps you need to consider your options. But just because you're going through fertility struggles doesn't mean that you *have* to do anything drastic career-wise. There's every chance you will get through it without making any career changes, so don't think it's an inevitability.

For example, Emma went through two rounds of IVF and everything that came before those, without making any drastic changes at work (OK, she probably stayed in one job longer than she would have, but that's no biggie).

Meanwhile, I decided to go freelance as I approached my IVF treatment. To be perfectly honest, I had been dreaming of doing that anyway and the upcoming treatment simply gave me a push. It did mean that I felt a lot less stress going into it, but I am a complete stress-head and tend to let work overwhelm me more than I really should – not everyone is like that. That decision had an impact on me when it came to maternity leave, but I wouldn't have had it any other way.

What's important is to not feel bad about any decision you make. The truth is, careers are longer than they ever were before, the idea of a job for life is gone, so over the course of your working life there are peaks and there are inevitable troughs. If you need to take your foot off the accelerator for a while, that is totally cool and you can absolutely put the pedal to the metal once you're ready again.

Employment rights – the facts

First, a very annoying fact: there is no statutory right for employees to get time off for IVF treatment. This is frustrating. It's the reason that those of us going through treatment generally don't take holidays, because you end up using all your days for various appointments and recuperation; however, employers should treat medical appointments related to IVF in the same way that they do any other medical appointment and shouldn't make you take a day off for little visits to the clinic.

Some employers are amazing and have fertility policies in place, including leave for treatment (more on this later). But they are few and far between. It's more likely that employers agree to flexible working arrangements or a combination of paid, unpaid, or annual leave during the treatment. Luckily, flexible working is becoming more prominent in most workplaces and shouldn't be a big deal for you to request. The chances are that you should be able to accommodate appointments within the boundaries of your working day.

If you're unable to work due to the effects of the treatment, employers should treat this sickness absence in the same way as sickness for other reasons. Likewise, if you have an unsuccessful round of IVF and need to stay on the couch, hide your puffy eyes, eat chocolate and watch *Homes Under the Hammer* for a few days, you have the right to sick leave. (Perhaps don't mention the chocolate and daytime telly part. In all seriousness you're grieving and coming to terms with something huge, you need time to recover.) Speak to your GP if you need a note.

Fact, less annoying: following a transfer, you are legally pregnant in the eyes of the law. We won't go into the emotional implications of this here, but once you've had a transfer, legally you're deemed pregnant and therefore you are protected from dismissal or adverse treatment under the Equality Act 2010 pregnancy legislation. This *does* require your employer's knowledge of the situation, so if you want to keep things quiet, you might not get this protection. But hopefully you won't find yourself in a position where it is needed. This protection lasts for two weeks after a negative test, or for the rest of the pregnancy if you get a BFP.

Fertility policies in the workplace (or the lack thereof)

Because, unlike maternity, there is no legal requirement for employers to offer anything to employees going through fertility treatment, very few have any sort of policy in place. This is annoying because people have literally nowhere to go to get info about how they will be treated without outwardly asking – and, as discussed, not everyone wants to do that, and to be frank, they shouldn't have to.

According to a study by Fertility Network UK and LinkedIn, only 26 per cent of people reported that their workplace had a policy relating to fertility treatment. With more awareness being raised all the time, this is expected to increase in the years to come, but for now, the chances are that your employer hasn't got anything down on paper when it comes to supporting you through treatment.

If you're feeling particularly strong and trailblazery today, you *could* approach your HR department and, if they don't have a policy, politely suggest that they create one. There are a number of resources for employers that you could point them in the direction of: namely Fertility Network UK and Fertility Matters at Work.

Here are a few examples of the fertility benefits offered by some employers, according to Fertility Network UK:

- Bristol City Council offers paid time off for fertility treatment granted to both partners (including same-sex partners) to attend one programme of treatment.

- Asda allows up to three periods of paid leave for
  IVF, with five days for women and one day for men,
  along with the option of swapping shifts to fit around
  appointments and additional unpaid leave if necessary.
  (Tesco offers something similar.)
- London & Quadrant Housing gives unlimited paid
  time off for fertility treatment!

Telling your boss

There comes a time in every person's infertility journey when it
would be helpful for bosses to know. This generally coincides
with treatment – the stress of lying about appointments and
trying to make excuses for nipping to the clinic really can make
an already shitty situation much worse. But it could also come at
a time when trying naturally is impacting your mental health and
you'd like the opportunity to explain what's happening to you.

That said, telling bosses isn't for everyone – and if that's you,
don't worry, you don't *have* to tell anyone. Fertility Network UK
did some research with LinkedIn and found that 62 per cent of
workers wouldn't discuss fertility issues with their employer, and
only 43 per cent of those undergoing treatment felt supported by
their boss. It's understandable not to want to mention it. But, with
the right boss, telling them what's going on can have its benefits.
Not least not having to lie every time you nip to the clinic.

I didn't mention it to mine until I had confirmed that I would
need treatment. I felt like going into a round of IVF without
letting her know would be more stressful than telling her. I was
very lucky in that my boss was an incredibly empathetic woman
with two children. I kind of knew she would take it well. Sure

enough, when I said I needed a quick word, took her into a meeting room and started to calmly tell her I would need IVF before bursting into messy, snotty tears, she was amazing. She also got emotional and told me I had her and the company's full support. Getting it out there really helped.

Here are a few points to note about telling the boss:

You decide how much to share

Just because you're letting your manager know that you're undergoing fertility treatment or struggling to conceive, this doesn't mean that they have to know *everything*. You only have to say as much as you feel comfortable with. To put a cap on any probing (we've all had enough of that, thank you) you could say something like, 'When I've got something to report, I'll let you know.'

Let them know what to expect

If this is the first time someone has told them about their fertility treatment, your manager might not have much idea of what it will mean for you and work. Again, this doesn't mean saying, 'I will have dildocam three times a week,' but you can outline that because of appointments you might need additional flexibility in your day.

You don't have to do it face to face

If busting into snotty tears in front of your boss (like I did) is a likelihood and you really don't fancy it, tell them over email. If you're writing it down, you can hit all the points you want to make and maintain your composure.

TTC when you're at the top of your work game

Sheila Cameron, CEO of Lloyd's Market Association, was working her way up in a male-dominated industry during her IVF struggle; now she advocates for more fertility support in the workplace: 'When my TTC journey started, my mother had just been diagnosed with terminal cancer. We had been trying for around 18 months and nothing had happened, and I had been trying to laugh it off, but I really wanted my mum to know we had got pregnant before she passed away, so we had tests done and started on the IVF treadmill. We were in the unexplained category, which used to drive me demented. I just kept thinking, it's only unexplained because you haven't done the right test yet!

'We tried a couple of IUIs: none of those worked. We moved to a new clinic and did more tests. Nothing was found. Did two rounds of IVF and both of those failed. We added some immuno-therapy and another round, which failed. At this stage, we had just had a BFN on the Friday, I called my dad to tell him and he burst into tears, because he knew my mum was hanging on to hear good news. I went home to see her before she passed away and spent about a month at home.

'When I got back to London, my appendix burst quite badly, and so I was off work for another month! I spoke to the IVF guys, who said that I couldn't do any treatment for three months. In that time I did a load of research about tests and realised that I hadn't had some basic blood-clotting investigations done. It turned out I had a blood-clotting issue.

'After four months of being off treatment, we did a fresh

round of IVF, with some blood thinners, and I got pregnant. I almost sailed through the start of the pregnancy, but at 11 weeks I had a massive bleed. After three years of treatment, that was the very first time my work found out that (a) I was pregnant; and (b) I had been doing IVF.

'I emerged from the bathroom in floods of tears and a colleague pulled me into a room (she had had a miscarriage the previous year), so I told her everything. She put me in a cab and sent me home. I rang my boss in the cab and told him everything. He was amazingly supportive, just fantastic, but shocked that all this had been going on and I hadn't told him.'

Keeping it quiet all that time

Shelia says, 'I work in the insurance industry, which is hugely male-dominated. There were very few women in senior positions and I thought I was better off not telling anyone. The reason we chose Guy's Hospital to begin with was that it was a 20-minute walk from my office. The reason we chose The Lister, when I switched clinics, was that they had a satellite office a five-minute walk from my office. I managed things so that I could get away with not telling anyone – choosing clinics that would help me to keep things hidden rather than ones that would be good for me.

'In hindsight, my boss couldn't have been more supportive. But I didn't want to have to tell everyone each time treatment didn't work. There were only a handful of people who knew what we were going through among our family and friends. When you have a negative you just want to crawl into a hole, eat a lot of pizza and drink a lot of wine. I couldn't cope with telling people and having to deal with their emotions as well – I struggled to deal with my own. I was also afraid that it would change how work saw me and my career prospects.

'There are two contradictory aspects to it: I didn't want them to know because they might put me in less challenging roles. On the flip side of that, I went and took roles where I wouldn't be too stretched. I guess I was protecting myself, and I was able to choose what would work for me; no one was making that choice for me. Later on, I did another round and got pregnant with twins. During that time, I took on quite a tough role, but it was one I knew was only for six to nine months because it was cover for someone else. I chose to put myself in that challenging position; if work had known I was trying to get pregnant, they probably wouldn't have put me in it. It was a control thing for me. I was making those decisions for me. And when you have so little control over your treatment and its outcomes – I needed control at work.'

Sheila has the following advice on fertility at work for employers and employees:

Tell your boss 'Now that I am a CEO, I actually go out and do talks about fertility at work, and I encourage women to tell their bosses and trust their manager. If your boss reacts badly, you're not in the right place, and you will probably get a bad response if you tell them you're pregnant, too.'

Know you're not alone 'One in six couples will struggle. I used to say to people that means there are probably at least two people on your floor going through the same as you. Don't think it's not happening, because it is!'

Employers: understand the value in support 'As an employer, if anyone is going through IVF I would want them to come and talk to me about it so that I could support them through it. What does that give me? It creates enormous loyalty and long-term support from that employee. I've seen it with people going through difficult pregnancies or adoption processes: what you get back in terms of loyalty is second to none. When I was going through treatment and my mum died, my appendix burst, and so on, I was with the same employer. I had to take so much time off. But they paid me throughout and never asked any questions. They supported me through one of my darkest periods, and I would have done anything for them.'

Host online support events 'It's about opening up the conversation. I recently did a talk at a company with two others also talking about their journeys, and that was facilitated online so that people could join anonymously. We said that no one has to put their name up or have the camera on.'

If you've been through it, speak up if you can 'Ideally, you need someone in leadership who has been through it and is willing to talk about it. Once one person opens up, more will generally follow. Standing up and speaking out makes it easier for others to come and talk to you and feel less alone – even if they decide not to share with their own boss. For me, being able to help people on a private one-to-one basis has been so satisfying.'

Conclusion

Dealing with infertility and your job at the same time is a real juggling act – one that occasionally means a few dropped balls. And that's OK – you're going through some big shit right here.

Balls and spinning plates aside, it's completely up to you how you choose to deal with work: whether you want to keep it all quiet or talk to your boss about what you're going through. Both options have their merits. We hope that this chapter has helped you as you navigate this tricky situation.

11

Pregnancy After Infertility and Loss

(Gabby)

Finally seeing those two little lines after any TTC struggle is a *big* moment. It's what you've been so desperate for, what you've dreamed about and why you danced under the full moon on a Tuesday for three months in a row. (What? You didn't try that? Slacker ...) Jokes aside, although this moment is one of unbridled joy, it can also come with its own baggage. You have got to where you wanted, but because of the journey to get you there, it can come with a bucket-load of anxiety that you just didn't see coming.

In this chapter, I will talk about the experience of being pregnant after infertility and loss, and hopefully give you some tools to get you through the next nine months (you're on your own after that – that's a different book).

What you'll find in this chapter:

- BFP – the first week.
- How hormones work in early pregnancy.

- Bleeding in early pregnancy and what can cause it.
- Cat Strawbridge on pregnancy after infertility.
- Meaningful milestones.
- Zoe Clark-Coates on pregnancy after loss.

'There are two lines!'

When we recorded a bonus episode of our podcast with three pregnant IVF-ers (Emma, Cat Strawbridge and Roma Agrawal), I was the only member of the conversation who wasn't, and never had been, pregnant. They were talking about the anxieties they all had and the parts of pregnancy they were finding tough. I remember sitting there thinking, 'You guys are crazy. Can't you just enjoy it?! If it were me, I'd be so happy all the time.' I just couldn't believe that achieving pregnancy wasn't the end of the struggle, until I found myself in that position, too, and realised that there are challenges in those nine months that follow.

I will say now, however, that the challenges of pregnancy after infertility, in my (and I think Emma's) experience, were nothing compared to the headfuck of trying, failing and not knowing whether it would ever happen for me. That was *much* worse. But still, it is worth talking about what happens next.

I was on cloud nine for at least a couple of weeks before the real challenges started. But there was one trigger moment on the day of my test when the little voice of doubt started to creep in. Having done the test at around 5am, I waited until it was a reasonable hour before calling the clinic to deliver the glorious news. I got through, told them I had a positive test and asked about getting enough drugs to get me through the 12 weeks until I could officially stop taking progesterone.

The nurse congratulated me and said that I only needed enough drugs to get me to my seven-week scan and, after that, assuming I was still pregnant they would give me enough for the 12 weeks. It was a pretty sensible point. They could give me what I needed after the scan. But the tiny amount of doubt that was cast – if I still needed the drugs after that or not – served to remind me that nothing was a given.

That was the start of my three-week wait. The wait that no one talks about. The one after your positive test until they are able to scan and see a heartbeat. I found it much, much easier than the other TWW, I was still high on a mix of relief and anticipation, but it was a thing. Many people find this one even harder than the first TWW, and it is not uncommon to get really addicted to peeing on sticks at this point, just checking that you're still pregnant. Every. Day. For me, I tested another two times and left it at that.

As it happened, I didn't have to wait for the full three weeks (more on that a bit later).

How hormones in early pregnancy work

Lots of people get quite hung up about the strength of a second line when they do a test. A strong line means loads of hCG; a weaker one less. But actually, individually, women have different levels of hCG in their system, so rather than the strength in one test, it's more important to focus on whether it gets darker over time.

The same can be said for blood tests, which will give you figures to do with hCG levels. One thing that is important to note is that women all have different levels of hCG, and might even have different levels themselves from pregnancy to pregnancy, so rather than focusing on the numbers, what is more important for doctors is that the amount doubles roughly every 48 to 72 hours.

Unless your clinic requests that you go for a blood test to confirm the positive test at home, there's a chance that you won't really experience the hCG levels headfuck. You'll just get a positive pee-stick (and a few more probably), then rock up for your first scan.

Your first scan

When people get pregnant naturally, their first scan will generally come at 12 weeks. If you're finally pregnant after a long time, but it was a natural conception, you're going to have to wait until 12 weeks, too (unless you cave and pay to have a private scan before then, which literally no one would blame you for doing).

When you've had fertility treatment, the chances are that your clinic will bring you in for a scan at seven weeks, so you'll get to see what's going on in there long before your fertile friends. Hurrah! A benefit for the infertiles! We'll take that, thank you very much. But before you get too excited, this early scan isn't really one you'd recognise from those pregnancy announcements you see on Facebook all the effing time. You really don't see a whole lot, but you will hopefully see a heartbeat. And that's quite exciting. You might also be able to see the gestational sac, the yolk sac and the foetal pole. Basically, a tiny circle, a bigger circle and a tiny little curved line. Most of these things will probably only be observed by the sonographer; you might just perceive a circle with a little flashing light.

If these things aren't observed, it's not the end of the world; they'll ask you to come back in about a week and check on things.

Why they do this scan

They sometimes do this scan with natural pregnancies, and it's usually to date the pregnancy. But of course, if you've had treatment you already have an accurate set of dates at your disposal. A fertility clinic will use this scan to establish a few things: the presence of a heartbeat (and how many heartbeats there are!), development of the embryo, and where it is (to rule out ectopic pregnancies).

Once they have done this, and assuming everything looks well, they will *discharge you from the clinic!* You don't get a graduation gown, just a surgical gown to wear during your last meeting with dildocam – but a graduation it is!

Then you're set free into the wild, like some sort of normal pregnant person. It's weird.

Bleeding in early pregnancy

I'm going to tell you the story about Harry the haematoma. I was working from home one day, I was around 6½ weeks pregnant and going about my day. I went for a quick wee and got the shock of my life. A big fat drop of deep red blood dripped into the toilet – it was so heavy I heard a plop. As you can imagine, I freaked out. I had heard about people bleeding in early pregnancy (Emma had already experienced it, too), but seeing such a large amount, it really didn't look as if things were OK.

I rang my clinic immediately and was told a nurse would call me back. After a long wait at my desk with my legs squeezed together to stop anything else from happening (side note: over 60 minutes = too long when you're losing your mind), I got a call from a nurse who offered to do a blood test if I came to the clinic, and I would get the results on Monday (it was Friday).

This felt entirely pointless. I needed to know *NOW* whether I was losing the baby. Casually waiting until Monday seemed outrageous. I ended up going to the clinic, because what else was I going to do? At first I was seen by the nurse, who unfortunately misread the room a little – not her fault at all – but she didn't really give me the reassurance I needed and spoke to me as if I was losing my pregnancy, offering gentle encouragement that I would have my baby one day. This set me off – serious water-works. She did the blood test, and as I was limping towards the exit, weeping, I asked if I could also speak to a doctor. I am so glad I did.

Thankfully, it was the doctor who had done my transfer and had clearly seen this many times before. He started by asking me to tell him exactly what was going on. He followed this up with reassurance that blood didn't have to be bad news. Then he offered me a scan. I had been told that there wasn't any point in a scan at six weeks because we probably wouldn't see a heartbeat anyway, but he said we might as well, because it *could* give us some clues.

The scan was great. We saw a heartbeat (the first time I had seen it!) and also a suspected area of bleeding, which looked like it could be a haematoma (explained below). Unfortunately, when the doctor pulled the probe out, it was covered in blood, as was the sheet on the chair I had been on. Again, he told me not to worry and as long as the bleeding stopped, it could all be fine.

I left feeling much, much better. It was very hard to reconcile seeing both a healthy-looking heartbeat *and* shit tons of blood, but a heartbeat there was, so I was able to function. Luckily, that night it all seemed to have passed (the blood that is). When the blood test results came in on the Monday, they showed healthy levels of hCG.

I had my seven-week scan booked in that Wednesday, so I got to see the heartbeat again, and this time the doctor confirmed that it was definitely a subchorionic haematoma. She booked me to go back and check it again at nine weeks and warned me that I might get a little more bleeding from the haematoma (by now christened, 'Harry' – by me, not the doctor). The hope was that it would be gone, or would have 'resolved' itself.

When I went back at nine weeks, it was still there, but it hadn't grown and no one seemed too bothered. It didn't come up again. End of the tale of Harry the haematoma.

Science bit: what is a subchorionic haematoma?

A subchorionic haematoma (or haemorrhage) is a little accumulation of blood between the amniotic sac and the wall of the uterus. It is one of the most common causes of bleeding in early pregnancy and is more common in IVF pregnancies. One particular study found that in a group of pregnant women, subchorionic haematomas developed in 22 per cent of the IVF group and in only 11 per cent in the non-IVF group.

Pregnancy after infertility: Cat Strawbridge

Cat Strawbridge, host of the Finally Pregnant podcast and event host, had three IUIs and six rounds of IVF (including two miscarriages) before she had her daughter, Wren. Here is her story: 'The round of treatment that gave us our successful pregnancy was really a case of "one more go for luck" due to our history and age: I turned 40 during that two-week wait. I went into the IVF transfer with a different frame of mind. I thought that if it's going to work, it's going to work – I couldn't take on any more than that. I was good, but I didn't use any of the alternative therapies I had previously and I didn't go organic, and so on. When it actually worked, it was a mixture of phew! And "Oh my God!"

'I did a test at around 3am and it was a faint line but inconclusive. We went into the clinic and for a blood test. Got a positive again. I decided to go in and do another blood test a few days later, too. We wanted to make sure that it was going the right way before we told anyone.

'The next few days and weeks I was a complete wreck. I rang the Early Pregnancy Unit at my local hospital and asked to go for an early scan because I couldn't wait until my scheduled early scan at seven weeks with my fertility clinic. They were really kind, and I must have been six weeks when we had our first scan and saw our first ever heartbeat. And then a second heartbeat. We couldn't believe it! We had transferred only one embryo, so it had clearly split. We didn't tell anyone it was twins initially, and then only shared the news with our families.

'In the first 16 weeks of my pregnancy, we had ten private scans in total – one every week or so. In one of those scans we found out that we had lost a twin. That was a different kind of shock. It took me a couple of days to get my head around it. I felt like we hadn't given "our little survivor" any attention during that scan, it was all about the loss, so we went for another scan to see her. I was a bit of a scan fiend.'

Scans

'I think you have to do what works for you. I learned that when I had scans booked in a couple of weeks away, the countdown started immediately. I realised it was better not to book them in advance, I'd rather book something at the last minute when I felt I needed to. It was easier, because otherwise it was all about looking ahead with anxiety.

'I think the scans were about the connection. You can't really connect when the baby is tiny – especially if you have been on a journey to get there. The scans help to fill that gap and let you know that there is something there.'

Enjoying

'I had started to enjoy the pregnancy, but the loss of the twin knocked me for six. Everyone was saying that it was a much safer pregnancy now because it was a singleton pregnancy after the loss, but I was still shaken. I remember when I was about 16 weeks and we had our family around for Christmas, I felt very conscious of my bump and I was still in a bit of denial and didn't want a fuss made of it. But I had started to believe that it could happen. Feeling movements at 18 weeks definitely helped to re-assure me, too. We had a thorough anatomy scan at that point and found out that we were having a little girl – that was a turning point for us, as we were really able to start bonding with her.'

Cat's advice for coping with pregnancy after infertility:

Put ego to one side

'Try to enjoy the pregnancy. The anxiety is real, but ask yourself – why not enjoy it? I quizzed myself on this repeatedly. And
ultimately, it came down to ego. If something went wrong, I
realised I was scared of being embarrassed for having enjoyed
it. Once I got that straight in my head and realised that my ego
shouldn't be a concern, I was able to let go of that. The reality
was, if something went wrong, I was going to fall, and fall hard.
It didn't matter if I had enjoyed it or not, so why not enjoy what
time I did have and hope it lasted?'

'Today I am pregnant'

'If looking ahead gets too much, bring it back to the present.
One of my phrases I suggest using is "Today, I am pregnant."
Someone texted me about this recently, saying that they had
used the mantra during their two-week wait even. They had
acted like, and imagined, that they were pregnant already.
Sadly, when she tested she got a BFN, but she said she had
enjoyed the TWW so much more because of it. She had that
time with her embryo. I love that, and it's how I tried to get
through my pregnancy.'

Step outside your comfort zone

'I really enjoyed pregnancy yoga, once I finally went along. I had
put it off and put it off because I was scared to admit that I was
pregnant, and I didn't want to jinx it – which is not possible and
totally down to mindset again. It was so nice to have put time
aside for me and my bump, and I wished I had gone sooner.

There was an element of feeling that I was the only infertile in the room, but I had to move past that.'

Getting support

'For most people, infertility doesn't leave you. I'm on a bit of a mission to ensure that the care people receive from their clinics continues into their pregnancy because you don't just stop needing support. And that's OK. Don't be surprised if you find yourself craving some TTC support in pregnancy, and don't be afraid to reach out if you do. I run the Finally Pregnant Hangout and other virtual events for people in this position.'

Your infertile-girl pregnancy milestones

Pregnancy can be a rollercoaster. Some days you're down. Some days you're up. Some days you feel anxious as hell. Some days you're filled with confidence and thinking about the future with excitement. But it's important to remember: you're going the right way. You're where you need and want to be. It's just that some days might be harder than others.

Milestone gifts

One of the really lovely things that Emma did to help me through my pregnancy was to buy me a little gift every four weeks. It was a tradition started by her best friend Sophie, who realised that Emma might need a little extra help enjoying her pregnancy (because of anxiety). Each month she bought her a gift to celebrate her progress. It was such a lovely idea that Emma did it for me, too. Some notable lovely things I received were: a banana protector (my craving was bananas, I know, it's bananas); a NARS lippie; some Neal's Yard Mother's Balm (hot tip for bumps).

If you circle this section of the chapter and leave it open when you see next your best mate, perhaps you'll get the same. Or casually mention this anecdote. Whatever works for you ...

Pregnancy has some fairly obvious milestones. Most of these are signalled with a scan, or by the advancement into a new trimester. These will definitely feel like achievements to arrive at. Here are just a few of the other, less obvious ones that we experienced and you might, too.

The first time you buy something

As with many things, this is different for everyone. Some people like to buy their future baby little things while they are still trying because it brings them hope. We have friends who bought baby grows each transfer. Some, like me and Emma, are too scared to even consider it. And, during IVF, they have long since stopped looking at baby clothes because it made them sad.

When you're finally pregnant, at some point you *will* be able to buy things! Buying your first thing is a nice moment. Whether it's an outfit or something for the nursery, it's nice. I waited until

20 weeks and splurged on an expensive outfit (Stella McCartney Kids, which, even though it was in the sale, was too much for a tiny tracksuit – but it made me very happy, so I guess it was priceless). Emma pretty much waited until her baby was born. I remember feeling quite nervous for her and the absence of any baby kit as her due date approached. But it all worked out. The baby wasn't naked for the first week or anything.

The first time you tell a stranger you're pregnant

Saying it out loud is a weirdly wonderful moment, too. You've probably told family and friends – so you've said it a few times. But how about a complete stranger? It came tumbling out of my mouth while I was ordering poached eggs at my favourite brunch spot. 'Can I have the eggs hard,* please – I'm, umm errr, pregnant ...' Eeeeekkkkk! I must have gone bright red, but I kind of loved it. Even though it came with a voice in my head saying 'Well, you've definitely jinxed it now.' But I told that voice to shut the f up because as we all know, *jinxing isn't real*.

The first time you look at a pregnant person and don't hate them

Now, this is a milestone you might never actually reach. Infertility does something quite strange to our brains when it comes to pregnant women. We have spent such a long time being triggered by them and feeling sad when we see them waddling around all fertile and smug that telling your brain 'It's OK now'

(*Side note – you don't need to eat your eggs hard any more, according to the NHS.)

doesn't always work. You'll live in this strange world where during antenatal appointments, NCT classes and pregnancy yoga classes you're surrounded by bumps, and it makes you uncomfortable, but you are one of them now. It's totally cool if you never actually feel comfortable around other preggos. It's just one of those symptoms of a TTC struggle. But there may come a day when you don't feel an instant pang of *eugh!* when you see them.

I think for me this was during my antenatal classes. I really liked my group, and I realised that it just didn't really bother me any more. They weren't smug preggos, they were just nice, somewhat terrified people in the same boat as me.

The first time you look pregnant

Oh, the bump. The thing you've longed for and dreamed of. *Where is it????* It turns out that bumps take a surprisingly long time to truly appear. And when you're feeling like a bit of a fraud, in a world of pregnant people that you don't feel comfortable around, having a bump becomes quite important for you.

I remember being so desperate to see the bump and feel pregnant, but it didn't really happen until after 20 weeks. Sure I had a small bump, but other people couldn't really see it (Emma was closer to 30 weeks before anyone noticed hers). Pregnancy yoga classes were where this really came to bear for me. I started them quite early, at about 14 weeks, when I didn't look pregnant at all. Cue serious imposter syndrome. I think it was at around 24 weeks and I was doing my yoga stretches and I was like 'Finally! I fit in!'

*The first time you make a list of names for your
actual baby*

Baby names are a big moment for us infertiles. It's something
we've been desperate to think about, but probably not going
there, for quite some time. If you're like me, you've watched other
people pop babies out and give their offspring names you were
hoping to use. *Arggghhhhhh!*

Now it's finally time to think of a name and, spoiler alert,
it's quite hard! When it's a real person, it makes baby names so
much more tricky. Starting to make a little list is a great moment,
although one often fraught with spousal disagreements, unless
you're going it alone, in which case it's just your own brain you
need to battle.

Pregnancy after loss: Zoe Clark-Coates

Having experienced the devastating loss of five babies in
pregnancy, Zoe Clark-Coates combined her heart-breaking
experience with her qualifications as a counsellor to write four
best-selling books, *Saying Goodbye*, *The Baby Loss Guide*,
Beyond Goodbye and *Pregnancy After Loss*. She is the CEO of
the global support charity the Mariposa Trust (widely known by
its primary support division Saying Goodbye) and she is co-chair
of the government's Pregnancy Loss Review Group on behalf of
the Health Secretary: 'Nothing could have prepared me for the
losses I suffered, but also nothing could have prepared me for
the trauma (and it was trauma) of pregnancy after those losses.

'Once you've had that trapdoor open and you've fallen, all the
innocence is taken from you, and you can't just presume that

everything is going to be OK. Suddenly you're living in trepida-
tion, fearing every day that something will go wrong. Your joy
is robbed – but there is also a lot of guilt involved. You want to
be able to enjoy it, embrace it and acknowledge that you're one
of the lucky ones – but at the same time, you're terrified – full of
fear, with no clue what tomorrow will bring.

'It is a battle with the mind to try to overcome that daily
anxiety, and nine months can feel like an eternity. I was blessed
because I used the tools from my training as a counsellor – skills
I had never intended to use on myself, but they became vital to
surviving each day.'

Here are a few of Zoe's top tips:

Telling people

'I'm a huge advocate for telling people you're pregnant as soon as
you feel ready. The 12-week rule is a not-so-subtle way of telling
people not to talk about loss. It's perfectly OK to wait until 12
weeks if that's what you want to do, but people shouldn't be
forced to conform to a rule that they never created. Some people
feel instantly ready to share the news, but they don't, as they fear
that they will be judged for sharing too soon.

'By telling your family and friends that you are expecting, you
enable those around you to support you through your pregnancy,
and if the worst does happen, they will be on hand to walk you
through a loss. The bottom line is that you should decide when
and who to tell, so be guided by your instincts and don't be
bound by society pressure.'

Give yourself space to worry

'We have all heard the advice "Take it one day at a time", which is solid guidance, but I am acutely aware that even 24 hours can feel too much for some people. To those people, I say take it hour by hour. Focus on the next 60 minutes in front of you, and remember that distraction can be a true blessing. Throw yourself into work. Spend time with friends and family. Take up a new hobby. The more you can immerse yourself into an activity, the less chance you have to worry and clock-watch.

'Allow yourself to feel what you feel. When people say, "I'm just not going to worry. I'm going to enjoy it," they can find themselves in a mental battle to keep negative thoughts at bay, and it is a clinically proven fact that the more you try not to think about something, the more your brain tries to take you there. So, actually, it can be a good practice to permit yourself to worry, but it's essential to limit the amount of time you give to it; for example, say to yourself, "I'm going to have five min-utes where I think about what is worrying me." I'll let my mind process the fear, and then at the end of the five minutes I will pull myself back and say, "I've given that worry the space to be heard, but now I rest on the truth that everything is OK, and my baby is safe."

'Remember, most of your worries have legitimate roots, and anyone with your experience could feel them. But the key is to not let yourself spiral down the path of "what-if", as it is long and never-ending! Make sure you pull yourself back into the current moment and hold on to the truth that right now, at this moment in time, everything is fine.'

You might experience what I call 'loo terror'

'Anyone who is pregnant following loss (and even some that have never gone through baby loss) will probably resonate with "loo terror". This is the term I named for the phobia of using the toilet in case you see blood. If you haven't ever experienced this, it's probably hard to grasp its magnitude, but it can be pretty debilitating.

'I remember so well how I would have to work up the courage to go to the loo, and at night I would give myself time off from looking and use the bathroom in the dark. At its worst, people drink less fluid so that they can reduce the number of loo visits. They avoid visiting places just in case they see red in public bathrooms, and they make themselves sore from constant wiping. Don't even get me started on recycled loo roll, as it often has red dots in it, and the panic from seeing those specks is enough to make you feel faint.

'The emotional effect of loo terror is significant, and people often feel that they are living on a knife edge in a constant state of anxiety. If you have experienced this, or are experiencing it, please know that you are not alone. This is 100 per cent common post-loss, and getting support can genuinely help. It is also common for this fear to continue on past pregnancy, and seeing blood during a regular monthly cycle can cause a similar psychological effect: heart pounding, panic, flashbacks, nausea, hot flushes, and so on. The first step to breaking the pattern is by talking about it. Know that what you are experiencing is sadly common, but help is available should you want or need it. '

Scan anxiety

'It is natural to find scans frightening after a previous pregnancy loss. My advice is always to be open about your history with whoever is looking after you. If you can explain what you have been through, they can tailor their support to your specific needs and requirements.

'Frustratingly, most women will see different clinicians each time they go for a scan, and retelling their story can be emotionally challenging and triggering, so I recommend writing a short note explaining your history and sticking it to the top of your maternity notes. Keep the note brief, as clinicians are often rushed, so sum up your story in as few words as possible, as this increases the likelihood of them reading it.'

Don't be afraid to change where you get your care

'In the UK, everyone can go to a different hospital or ask for another doctor/midwife to be in charge of their care. If you find specific places or people triggering, definitely request a change. We cannot control so much in pregnancy, but who looks after us and where we get seen is within our power to alter.'

Conclusion

It's the ultimate aim of TTC, but pregnancy comes with its own baggage, and many of us really haven't dared to consider what happens when we see those two little lines. What should you expect to happen next? How will it all play out? We hope we've given you some idea of what might go down once you've cried those happy tears while wielding a plastic stick covered in your own wee.

Importantly, pregnancy can be an anxious time for any woman – for someone who has struggled to get to that point, or has sadly lost a pregnancy before, it can be a very difficult period, filled with fear and a whole boatload of other emotions. But you can get through it and maybe even start to enjoy it (or even just parts of it).

We also hope this chapter has offered some comfort in hearing the stories of others and perhaps even given you some tools to make the pregnancy easier.

12

Pregnancy Loss and Dealing with Grief

(Emma)

Let's start this most difficult of chapters with a cold, hard statistic: a quarter of pregnancies end in loss. That isn't, I imagine, any help at all if you have recently experienced it, particularly if it was a longed-for baby. The reality is that pregnancy loss is one of society's last taboos, and to that end people tend to be very dismissive about it. Therefore, not only are those grieving the loss of their baby likely to be grappling with the emotions surrounding it, but they also might find their grief is dismissed by those around them, which makes the whole situation even harder.

The way people experience pregnancy loss – just like the way people experience pregnancy, or infertility, or anything, really – differs from person to person. Some are able to dismiss it as an inconvenience; for others, it is crushing. If you are reading this book and have lost a pregnancy, I imagine that you are in the latter camp: you might have lost a baby you conceived after years of trying, or you might have experienced recurrent losses.

Some more stats: according to Tommy's (the pregnancy

charity) the overwhelming majority of pregnancy losses happen in the first 12 weeks of pregnancy, with about 2 per cent of pregnancies resulting in a 'late miscarriage' during the second trimester (after 24 weeks, the death of a baby is called a stillbirth).

About 1 per cent of women in the UK will experience recurrent pregnancy loss (that's more than three in a row, although campaigners are trying to reduce this to two), whereas six in ten of those who experience recurrent losses will eventually go on to have a successful pregnancy.

We've put grief and pregnancy loss together in the same chapter because we want to make it clear that even though you might not have experienced a pregnancy loss in the 'traditional' sense, that is, after a positive pregnancy test, the emotions around different types of loss can be similar, whether it's a pregnancy you knew about or a child in mind. That's because grief isn't always about losing a baby: it's about losing a future. While the first section of this chapter is about the practical side of pregnancy loss and what you might experience, the second half is about the emotional side and how to manage the grief you experience after a child that you have called into being doesn't make it earthside.

What you will find in this chapter:

- The language of loss.
- What is pregnancy loss? The different types of loss and why they happen.
- Signs that you are experiencing a pregnancy loss and what to do about it.
- What to expect during a pregnancy loss.
- Managing your pregnancy loss.
- What happens next: grief.

- You're not mad. Why we mourn people we have never met.
- Some ideas for dealing with grief.

Yet another note on language

The language around a lot of gynaecology is problematic, but nowhere more so than when it comes to the loss of a pregnancy. From the outdated term 'spontaneous abortion' to the phrase 'incompetent cervix', the language used around pregnancy loss has always tended to assign blame to the woman. The very condition of being a woman already makes us feel guilty enough about almost everything; we don't need the words our doctors use to make us feel even worse. 'Miscarriage' is one of those terms; the mis- suffix connotes a mistake. When Hillary Clinton famously 'misspoke', it was she who had got the facts wrong. A 'misstep' is when you make a blunder. To 'mislead' someone is to tell a lie. In all cases, the subject has done something wrong. As we will find out in this chapter, miscarriage is almost never the subject's fault, which is why we have chosen to use the term 'pregnancy loss' throughout this book.

The good news is that the language is beginning to change as obstetrics evolves, but those attitudes are still lingering among clinicians who have been practising for a few decades.

What exactly is pregnancy loss?

The clinical term 'miscarriage' is the spontaneous end of a pregnancy before 23 weeks and six days' gestation. It's important to define it properly before we start, to make clear that it is *spontaneous*: it's no one's fault. As with all things infertility, pregnancy loss isn't straightforward: there are many types.

Chemical pregnancy is an 'early' pregnancy loss that occurs around the five-week mark. You might have had a positive pregnancy test but no symptoms of pregnancy yet. The symptoms tend to be some spotting, mild abdominal cramping and then a heavier-than-usual period. If you have a blood test to confirm your pregnancy (after IVF, for example), it will show low hCG levels. Don't let the dismissive terminology prevent you from treating this type of pregnancy loss with the gravity it deserves: your baby, however small, has died. If you are feeling grief, it is completely legitimate.

Missed miscarriage occurs when a pregnancy seems to be progressing normally, with the full complement of head-in-toilet, beige-food-only symptoms, but a scan indicates that there is no heartbeat or the baby has stopped growing. Essentially, your body hasn't caught up with the baby yet and begun to end the pregnancy. We'll cover what happens next further on in the chapter.

Blighted ovum is another type of missed pregnancy loss, this is also known as an anembryonic pregnancy. This happens when the embryo stops developing very early on, but the sac that would contain it continues to grow, so you continue to experience symptoms. This is usually discovered at a scan, which shows there is no 'foetal pole' (the beginnings of the foetus).

Ectopic pregnancy If you thought the grief and shock that comes with pregnancy loss was already unthinkable, with an ectopic

pregnancy it might also be life-threatening. An ectopic pregnancy, which occurs in about 2 per cent of pregnancies, happens
when the embryo implants somewhere outside the womb, usually
the Fallopian tubes. Sometimes the baby stops developing and is
reabsorbed into the body. If it continues to grow, though, your
tube might rupture, which will need urgent medical attention.
If you have crippling abdominal pain or pain in your shoulders,
see a doctor straight away.

Molar pregnancy This is extremely rare. A molar pregnancy,
also known as a hydatiform mole, happens in one in 600 pregnancies. There are two types: a complete molar pregnancy and
a partial molar pregnancy. In the former, there is no foetus at
all – instead, the placental tissue develops into fluid-filled cysts.
In a partial molar pregnancy, some normal placental tissue might
form along with the abnormal tissue, and a foetus might also
form, but it won't be able to survive. This will be detected at the
first scan at around 12 weeks and confirmed with a blood test;
molar pregnancies often emit much higher hCG than usual.

In a few cases, a hydatiform mole can develop into cancer.
According to the Miscarriage Association, about one in ten
women who are diagnosed with a molar pregnancy require
chemotherapy, although the charity also points out that treatment is close to 100 per cent effective and almost never harms
your chances of having children in the future.

We've covered the types of pregnancy loss, but why do they
happen? The chances are very high that everyone from your
doctor to your best friend will point out that it's 'just one of
those things' or it 'wasn't meant to be', but actually, there are a
number of very real reasons why they occur.

The reasons for pregnancy loss

Chromosomal problems Chromosomes are the building blocks of life that control everything from eye colour to hair thickness. Sometimes the developing foetus gets too many (or not enough) chromosomes and can't develop any further. Unless you or your partner has a chromosomal disorder, such as Mr Emma's Robertsonian translocation, this tends to be a random, one-off occurrence. If you have had three or more losses, a recurrent miscarriage clinic might want to test the remains of your baby for abnormalities.

Hormonal problems Your body's production of hormones, particularly progesterone, oestrogen and TSH, the thyroid hormone, can affect your ability to carry a baby to term, which is why they are checked when you are undergoing initial fertility tests. Recently, two major trials have provided some evidence that offering women who have experienced recurrent pregnancy loss progesterone supplements might increase their chances of keeping a pregnancy.

Blood clotting issues Some conditions, such as Hughes syndrome, make the blood 'sticky' and prone to clotting, making it harder for blood vessels to supply the placenta. This is not detected by routine fertility tests, but it should be tested for at a recurrent miscarriage clinic.

Illness This includes STDs such as chlamydia and bacterial vaginosis, but it also includes illnesses such as malaria, rubella (which is why we vaccinate against it), and even some types of food poisoning.

Anatomical problems We've covered fibroids and abnormally shaped uteruses elsewhere in the book (on pages 76 and 77): both can affect your ability to carry a baby to term. In addition to those is a weakened (*never* 'incompetent') cervix, which can be caused by procedures such as the removal of pre-cancerous cells around your cervix and cause pregnancy loss. Midwives tend to be fairly hot on this and will check the state of your cervix at each scan. Weak cervixes can be treated with cerclage procedures, also known as a cervical stitch, or an abdominal suture, which is higher up in the cervix.

Signs you are experiencing pregnancy loss and what to do

Take it from us: if you have been through any kind of infertility, early pregnancy in particular is not going to be an easy ride. After the initial high of the BFP subsides, the slightest twinge or a few hours of relief from the symptoms of pregnancy might cause you to panic and, if you are anything like us, instantly start googling 'early pregnancy units open at the weekend' (these things *always* happen at the weekend).

Kate Marsh is the midwifery manager at Tommy's, the pregnancy charity. She says the two most obvious signs that you might be experiencing pregnancy loss are pain and bleeding. This varies by person and gestation. 'You might just get some spotting or you might get some quite heavy bleeding straight away, or anything in between. With the pain it might start off as period-type pains and then increase from there. Others might get sudden pain that happens quite quickly.'

Bleeding, though, happens fairly frequently in early pregnancy:

it could be hormonal (some women continue to get monthly 'periods' early on in pregnancy, whereas others, like me, simply have an overly dramatic cervix that bleeds at the slightest sign of trouble) or it could be something else: both Gabby and I had a fairly harmless condition called a subchorionic haematoma at the beginning of our pregnancies (explained on page 226), which studies have suggested is more prevalent in IVF pregnancies. Bleeding alone, then, is not necessarily a sign that you are losing your baby.

Loss of symptoms can be another indicator, although, again, even during the first trimester, pregnancy symptoms tend to ebb and flow. Women who have experienced a pregnancy loss often mention a hunch or an instinct that tells them this is what is happening, although this is sometimes hard to separate from common or garden anxiety, particularly if this is a longed-for baby.

Kate's advice is that if you are experiencing severe pain or any kind of bleeding, you should head straight to your nearest early pregnancy unit (EPU) if it accepts self-referrals or A&E if not, or contact your GP if you are clinically stable. If you are still in the first few weeks of your pregnancy, they will take your blood to measure the amount of hCG and progesterone and might scan you to see if they can find the baby (although before about six weeks it might be too small to find, even on an internal ultrasound).

The reason for this urgency is that they will want to ensure you are not experiencing the first signs of an ectopic pregnancy, which needs immediate medical attention.

Line eyes: why your POAS obsession isn't helping

Internet forums are awash with women obsessing over the colour of the line on their 'pee on a stick' (POAS) pregnancy test: 'Is today's darker than yesterday's?' 'Does it look like it's fading?' 'Shouldn't it say "3 weeks +" by now?'

Don't be tempted to join the ranks of those obsessing over pregnancy tests. It isn't worth it. Pregnancy tests only measure the concentration of hCG in your urine at a given moment. Even if you're using 'first-morning urine', the amount of water you had last night or the number of times you went to the loo in the middle of the night will have an impact on the colour of the line. What looks like a fading line progression could easily be happening because you're just ultra-hydrated today.

The only way to properly confirm that your hCG levels are progressing as they should be is to get a blood test, either from your clinic if you have undergone fertility treatment, or an early pregnancy unit if you haven't and are concerned. We've even heard of podcast listeners who have persuaded their GP to do a test for them.

We've all been obsessive pregnancy test takers. If you get that elusive BFP after years of trying, it can be so unbelievable that the temptation is often to keep making sure that it's still there – and if you've previously had a loss, it can be soothing to keep checking. But repeated POASing can also cause unnecessary misery, so if you are lucky enough to get a BFP, take a test, then perhaps

use the second one in the box to confirm it. Do one the
following week if you're worried that your symptoms
are off. But, for the love of everything that is good and
holy, don't keep doing them every day. It isn't worth
the anxiety.

What to expect during a pregnancy loss

Pregnancy loss is such an under-discussed subject that many
women who go through it are surprised by the physical symptoms they experience, let alone the emotional anguish that comes
with it. Because of the way it is referred to in hushed tones, or
depicted on TV (ahem, *Fleabag*), most women expect pregnancy
loss to involve a bit of bleeding on the toilet while a single tear
slides tragically down their face. The medical community doesn't
always help: lots of our podcast listeners were told by their doctors 'It'll be just like a slightly heavier period.' But in many cases,
it's more complicated than that. Here are some things you might
not know that you'll experience:

It might be heavier than a 'heavy period' Lots of women report
that what they experienced is a lot more painful and involves a
lot more blood, although occasionally everything is reabsorbed
and there isn't much bleeding. As with everything, it depends on
your body. In most cases, though, the likelihood is that at some
point the bleeding will be so heavy that the only place you can
comfortably sit is on the toilet. Once it has abated a little, you
can use pads (don't use a tampon).

Contractions Even during early pregnancy losses, your uterus is working hard to push out the tissue associated with the pregnancy: the lining, the placenta and your baby. The cramps, or even contractions, may be intense and go on for hours, and you might even feel the urge to push. One of my friends, who lost her baby at ten weeks, described it as going through a 'mini-labour', while those who have experienced later losses, after around 15 weeks, say what they experienced was similar to full labour.

There will be clots During an ordinary period, your body spends two weeks building up a lining and shedding it. If you're experiencing pregnancy loss, that lining has been accumulating for *weeks*, so expect to pass very large clots, and lots of them. Before about ten weeks, the tissue you pass will look a bit like liver, whereas after about ten weeks it might be more jelly-like as the placenta forms.

You might see your baby Even at six weeks, the baby is the size of the nail on your little finger. Some women report feeling an urge to touch or even photograph their baby, no matter how small, whereas some choose to keep the remains of their baby and bury it.

You might keep bleeding for weeks The main event will probably take place over the course of a few hours or a couple of days, but because your body has a lot of tissue to get rid of, the chances are you'll keep bleeding for two or three weeks after you have lost your baby. It might even last longer; some people report their spotting continued for three months after their loss. This is your body expelling the last of your pregnancy tissue – don't use a tampon.

You'll feel physically ill Going through 'mini-labour' and losing a lot of blood will take it out of you, and you might feel exhausted, sick, dizzy and weak for a few days after the main event is over. Be kind to yourself; work can live without you for a few days.

Your hormones will crash During your pregnancy, your oestrogen, progesterone and hCG levels have been climbing fast, with your hCG level doubling every two days. In the days after you lose your pregnancy, they will come crashing down. Again, be gentle with yourself. You might experience symptoms such as tiredness, anxiety, depression, irritability or even insomnia, and that's without factoring in the emotional trauma of loss.

In later pregnancy, you might go through a full labour. After 12 weeks, you might feel a rush as your waters break; after 16 weeks it's likely you'll need to stay in hospital while a specialist midwife talks you through labour. Sometimes this will be on a labour ward, although in other hospitals it might be on a gynae ward.

One of the most cruel things your body does if your baby dies after about 16 weeks is to lactate; yes, your milk may come in. That means that while you are grieving the loss of your child, your body is reminding you what you've lost with hard, swollen, sore and leaky breasts. Your midwife should be able to explain how to manage this and prevent mastitis. Some women choose to pump and donate their milk to a milk bank. Others pump and bury it with their baby, while others still just want it to go away as soon as possible. It goes without saying that any decision you make is a completely valid response to grief.

Managing your pregnancy loss

One of the hardest parts of this is the routine way in which many clinicians treat pregnancy loss. Thus, as you are still reeling from being told you have lost your baby, it's likely your doctor will probably offer you one of three ways to proceed:

Expectant management

This is the term given to 'going home and waiting for it to happen naturally'. Most doctors recommend this option if you are in your first trimester and your pregnancy loss looks fairly 'straightforward' – even if it's ectopic but doesn't seem life-threatening. Stock up on painkillers (the stronger, the better), sanitary pads (be warned: the largest, most absorbent pads available are marketed as 'maternity pads') and give yourself a break – now is not the time to put pressure on yourself because you aren't hitting your daily 5k target.

Also be prepared to wait. After a missed miscarriage, it could be a couple of weeks before your body catches up and the process begins in earnest. Psychologically, those weeks can be excruciating.

If you choose this option, you might be asked to take a home pregnancy test a few weeks after the pregnancy ends to make sure that your hCG levels have dropped back. You should also be offered a scan if your bleeding and pain haven't subsided within a couple of weeks.

Medical management

The second option is to take a drug called misoprostol, either in pill or pessary form. Although most doctors will recommend expectant management first, you have the option to insist on a medically managed miscarriage; some people just want it to be over. In other cases, the doctor might advise you to take this option if you have been waiting for a missed miscarriage to happen for more than two weeks.

There are downsides to this option. Misoprostol causes uterine contractions (that mini-labour again). A lot of our podcast listeners say that they were surprised by the severity of the pain (although some were surprised by the lack of pain, so it varies), and the cramps might continue for up to a week, so stock up on painkillers. There are also side effects, including diarrhoea and vomiting (to add to the dignity of the occasion).

Sometimes you might be asked to stay in hospital overnight, or you may have to return if the bleeding doesn't start within a day or if it is very heavy. You may also be asked to hover over a cardboard bedpan when you go to the loo so that your doctors can be sure you have passed the full placenta. That means, depending on your gestation, it is very likely that you will see your baby, which can be traumatic.

In some cases the pills don't work and you need to take them again. Misoprostol works about 85 per cent of the time. If it's an ectopic pregnancy but doesn't seem life-threatening, you might be offered a drug called methotrexate, which comes in injection form, instead.

Surgical management

Sometimes, if expectant management hasn't worked or a scan has shown that there is 'retained tissue' (no, we don't love that term either), or if you just want this to be over right now, your doctor might suggest surgical management, also known as a D&C (dilation and curettage), ERPC (evacuation of retained products of conception) or SMOM (surgical management of miscarriage).

This can take place under local or general anaesthetic. The procedure is usually the same for both: the cervix is dilated, then a suction tube is used to remove the tissue (obviously, if you're under local anaesthetic, you'll also get a *lot* of painkillers). It usually takes about ten minutes. There are risks associated with some of the methods of surgical management: very occasionally it can cause scarring to the uterus, known as Asherman's syndrome, so it's worth having a conversation with your doctor before you make any decisions.

Some women report that this option was the easiest for them: it was over and done with quickly and the recovery time is relatively speedy. On the other hand, some said going through the physical process of passing their baby helped them come to terms with their loss. It's also worth bearing in mind that you can request that the surgeon keeps your baby for you to bury.

Amy's story

Amy Culpin lost three pregnancies – two IVF and one natural – over the course of 14 months. She now has a daughter, Freya, who was born in early 2021. 'All my losses were very different.

The first one was after my second embryo transfer – we'd had a BFN on the first go. We presumed everything was fine until the viability scan. Then we went in and they said, "There is something there, but we can't see a heartbeat. We'd like to see that by now, but come back next week, it might just be too early." That first time, I was so naive to it. I thought: *OK, I'll come back next week and everything will be fine.*

'In the meantime, though, I started bleeding and miscarried naturally. Everything took me by surprise. I'd had spotting for a few days, then there were two or three really intense hours. I didn't know what to do. When you lose a pregnancy in a toilet, it's down to you to deal with it. My options were: take it out of the toilet – and do what? – or flush it. I found that really hard; there's no right or wrong.

'That miscarriage happened on 23 December. That Christmas we went out for dinner with my parents and the people on the table next to us were doing a pregnancy announcement. I just thought: *Why us? Why is this happening to us?*

'After that, I had one failed embryo transfer, and another where I transferred two embryos and got a positive on test day. The tests were really odd: in the afternoons they were really strong, in the mornings they were really weak. When we went for the viability scan, there was one sac but nothing in it. I didn't even have a massive bleed with that; I just had spotting. Those were our last two embryos, so as well as grieving the pregnancy, we were grieving the fact that six embryos had amounted to nothing.

'In some ways, the third loss was the worst, because it was so dragged out, although because it was a natural pregnancy I felt in many ways that it was too good to be true. I'd had a bit of a bleed so we went for a scan at the early pregnancy unit. I think

I was six weeks at this point. Similar to the first one, they said: "There is something there, but it's smaller than we'd like to see, so come back next week." So I went back at seven weeks, and it was the same thing: "It's grown, but it's still not as big as we'd like. Come back next week." This went on from six to ten weeks. The uncertainty was awful. I knew deep down it wasn't going to be viable, so I said, "Can you just call it? Can you just tell me that this is not a viable pregnancy, then give me a D&C so it's over?" They wouldn't call it; they said, "Sorry but we have to keep checking. Your dates might be wrong."

'At ten weeks, the day before my appointment, I started bleeding. I was at work in the daytime and I went to the toilet and saw I was bleeding. That evening I had a feeling: I knew it was about to start coming away. I was having dinner and I suddenly felt like I was going to pass out. I just knew I needed to be on the toilet, because something was about to happen. I think I passed it around 8pm. This one was the worst, pain-wise: although the embryo was really small, the sac wasn't. Now I've been in labour, I know I was having contractions, I had to push it out.

'No one talks about the physical side of miscarriage: it's painful, it hurts. The third one happened on a Tuesday, and for the rest of the week I just stayed in bed, partly because I was crying so much, but partly because I was physically just exhausted. You go through so many emotions.

'When it came to my pregnancy with my daughter, I was a wreck. Even giving birth, I was constantly asking if she was OK. That's the terrible thing about pregnancy loss: no one tells you that it's going to be all-consuming.'

Grief

Pregnancy loss can be a terrible physical and emotional experience, but grief can come at any stage of TTC. It doesn't matter where you are – whether you're still in the monthly cycle of hope, pregnancy test, grief; or you've lost a pregnancy or a baby; or you've had a failed round of IVF – that all-encompassing sadness you're experiencing which you can't seem to move on from – that's grief.

Some people manage to move through it quickly, whereas others need help dealing with it. This section will look at why we experience grief during TTC and will offer some tips on coping with and working through it.

Why we grieve people we've never met

The rest of this chapter will address grief and why it's important to accept that you are grieving, even if you haven't experienced what other people might term a 'loss'. To help us through this difficult time, allow me to introduce Julia Bueno, a psychotherapist and counsellor who specialises in miscarriage and infertility, and whose book, *The Brink of Being*, is essential reading for anyone who has experienced pregnancy loss, which includes the loss of what she calls 'a child in mind'.

Julia is one of the most articulate people around on the subject of pregnancy loss. She has a knack of putting into words those feelings that had, until she described them, been loose, unformed thoughts floating around the outer reaches of your brain. A conversation with her will (a) involve dozens of moments where you squeal 'Oh my *God*! That's *completely* how it feels!'; and (b) take *hours*, due to the frequency with which you are interrupting her to make point (a).

One of her central points is that loss can come at any stage of pregnancy – even before a positive pregnancy test – because of the relationship we develop with the 'unborn'. She uses the term 'a child in mind', a concept she has borrowed from author Hilary Mantel to mean an unborn baby with whom you have developed a bond. It doesn't matter how fleeting its existence was: whether it was early gestation, at embryo stage or even wasn't ever actually conceived. What matters is that you 'called the child into being' and developed a relationship with it, which means when it, or the possibility of it, is gone, you grieve it: 'A woman calls her pregnancy into whatever state it wants to be,' says Julia. 'For some women, it might be a cluster of cells until such time she calls her child into being.

'Biology might say and ethics might say and law might say a child doesn't come into being until x. But this is not what we're talking about. This is an incredibly powerful bond with a child that lives in an imagination. And our imaginations are super-powerful things: they reorganise our brains and cause body states and cause hormones and neurotransmitters to be released and stopped. They have profound effects on our heart and our body systems. Do not underestimate the power of our imagination.'

The bond with the child that didn't happen is 'profound and nuanced', she adds. So when you feel that sense of loss and sadness after a pregnancy loss or negative pregnancy test, make sure you treat it as the grief it is.

My story

The months running up to my first frozen embryo transfer were surprisingly fraught, considering how 'relaxed' I was trying to be. After my egg collection in September, we had to wait until the end of my cycle for the results of the PGD, then I had to have a month on the Pill before I began the meds for the transfer. By the time we got to embryo transfer time, it was late November and I thought that I would *die* of impatience. Honestly, until transfer day, it hadn't really crossed my mind that it might not work. We had had a textbook egg collection, with a staggering five embryos being given the all clear after PGD testing. As soon as I had my embryo on board, I gave myself free rein to imagine what it would be like if this little thing turned into a real baby. Internet message boards had taught me the term 'PUPO', but as everyone around me pointed out: 'Why *wouldn't* it work? There's no point in worrying.'

Mr Emma and I drove to Cornwall and stayed in a little chalet looking out over the sea for the first week of the two-week wait and sat up at night playing Scrabble next to the wood-burning stove, talking about baby names and nursery colour schemes. During the day we wandered on the beach or went on trips to beauty spots and had arguments about schooling options. I have a photo of myself on a rope bridge at the Eden Project trying not to look cross that Mr Emma wouldn't even *discuss* single-sex education.

Test day was done by the book: waiting the full 11 days (my reasoning: nothing can go wrong if you follow instructions correctly). I even used the test the clinic had provided me with: a cheap one with a fuzzy blue control line. It was negative. I couldn't understand it: *I had seen the embryo go in.* I couldn't even get pregnant when a healthy embryo was physically put inside me.

We went back to bed and held each other and I sobbed until my face was raw. Every now and then a new thought would wash over me and I'd start sobbing again: 'I'm going to have to go through this whole hideous process again.' 'I'm going to be going through it for years.' 'I'm never going to have a baby.' 'My arms are so empty. I need something small and wriggling on my lap, and I need it *now*!'

I somehow transferred myself to the sofa and texted my mum to say it was negative, then I couldn't bring myself to answer the phone because I felt so ashamed. I had been talking to anyone who would listen about this: everyone had got their hopes up and I had failed them. My sister showed up on my doorstep with a poinsettia (it was Christmas) and a box of Lindor, then climbed onto the sofa and hugged me while I sobbed.

The following few days were a blur: I dragged myself into work and told my boss and continued to feel ashamed. He – an empathetic soul – said how sorry he was, then spent the rest of the meeting complaining about his infant daughter.

We hosted a Christmas party for my friends and their kids and I tried to look cheery.

We got a cat.

At the end of that week I went to my office knees-up, where I demanded that my boss buy me a bottle of champagne, sank it, then marched up to a colleague who reported to me, and forced him, using my epic sixth sense for people who are knocked up, to admit his wife was pregnant. 'We haven't told anyone yet,' he mumbled. 'Her family has a history of miscarriages, so we want to keep it quiet.' 'Pffft!' I slurred. (Note: I have subsequently apologised, offered a full explanation of my appalling behaviour and begged for forgiveness. He is a very nice man and is OK with it.)

I felt guilty for not being able to get on with life. It was an embryo, for God's sake – a cluster of cells. It had no human characteristics. It was a tiny blob, invisible to the naked eye. What gave me the right to feel so sad? There were women out there who had seen their babies' hearts beating, or had seen a tiny, perfectly formed hand on a scan, or who had felt them kick or *reached full term* and then lost their babies. *They* were allowed to experience grief. *I* was sad because of … nothing. No bleeding, no particular symptoms, just two weeks and then a negative pregnancy test. The absence of a line. It was just like all the other tests I had taken. What gave me the right to have such strong emotions?

Obviously, I now know that I was experiencing grief. The fact that I didn't feel able to mourn probably made it worse: not only was I really, really sad, but also I didn't feel that I had the right to my sadness. The problem was that there was no event I could point to – it was an absence of an event. Grotesquely, I found myself wishing that I had had a pregnancy loss, just so that I could have something to point to which people would understand. It was a weird, twisted emotional place to be.

It's not your fault

Because it is inside our bodies that the pregnancy, or lack thereof, has happened, a lot of us automatically blame ourselves if we can't conceive or we lose a pregnancy, but of course it *isn't* your fault. Unless you have spent a couple of weeks merrily bodybuilding, ingesting industrial-grade chemicals and repeatedly punching yourself in the stomach, it's very, *very* unlikely that anything you did contributed to the reason you are grieving.

Julia says that there are two reasons why we tend to blame ourselves: firstly, old-fashioned misogyny and its effect on society, which shames women for not being able to produce children. Secondly, our existential need to seek out explanations for things that don't make sense. 'What do we do as human beings but fill in the gaps?' says Julia. 'We say, "It must be me. I've been told we don't know [why], but I'm going to have to come up with a reason. My prefrontal cortex will try to come up with a reason."'

It's 'making sense of not knowing', she says. Your job, as the person who is grieving, is to repeatedly explain to yourself that *it is not your fault*. If the self-blame becomes really bad, seek help. 'Part of therapy is getting us as human beings to sit with the not knowing,' says Julia. 'We have to sit with the fact that we are little creatures on this earth and random shit happens.'

Dealing with grief

It seems silly for me to try to cover something as vast and all-encompassing as dealing with grief in one small section of a book, but here I go anyway.

Julia says that part of the reason we don't recognise what we are going through during infertility or after pregnancy loss as 'grief' is because you can't pin down what you are grieving. 'It's this sort of inchoate grief of a future,' she says. 'You can't hold on to it, as opposed to grief of a human being who lived and breathed on earth. That's something a little bit more tangible.'

Here are some ways to help you grieve:

Accept your grief

The point about grief for infertility is that it's happening, whether you recognise it as such or not. And it's usually cumulative: either you are experiencing it each month when you see a negative pregnancy test, or you had built up hope that *this was your time* and it has all come crashing down with a pregnancy loss.

Some people experiencing infertility or loss (and most unhelpful friends and relatives) automatically go into 'at least' mode: 'At least I wasn't very far along', 'At least I know I can get pregnant', 'At least I'm not like Barbara over the road, with that funny wart on her forehead.' That sort of reaction isn't helpful because it invalidates your feelings. Give yourself permission to mourn.

Understand your grieving style

You've probably heard about the stages of grief: shock and denial; pain and guilt; anger and bargaining; depression, reflection and loneliness; the 'upward turn'; reconstruction; and, finally, acceptance (there's a great *Simpsons* episode in which Homer goes through all of them in 20 seconds, google it). But the reality is that, as Julia points out, everyone does it differently. Not only will you grieve differently from your friend who has also had a baby loss, but you and your partner are likely to experience it in different ways, too.

Julia talks about 'instrumental' and 'intuitive' grieving styles. She attributes them to males and females but points out that this is a 'blunt instrument' to describe people's grieving styles: 'I would say that I'm a very male griever, I'm a very instrumental griever.'

Instrumental grieving is the name given to those who get up and 'do'. They tend to be men. 'They might look like they're coping quite well, because they're running a marathon or they're cleaning up the loft or they're being very practical organising the funeral,' she says. 'I spoke to a woman who has been running a helpline for years and she says that it is the men who will call up and say, "I had a stillbirth last week – can I sign up for the marathon?"'

She says a common mistake is to assume that instrumental grievers aren't upset. 'Just because somebody's running a marathon doesn't mean that they're not feeling the loss in an equally powerful, profound way as somebody who is sitting in a corner, crying.'

Intuitive grieving is the more traditional version, which tends to be regarded as a more female way of feeling loss. 'Bereavement literature says that women tend to grieve outwardly, expressing their emotions and using networks, leaning on loved ones.' Both are an equally acceptable way of feeling loss, she says.

Find a way to tell your story

Because the world finds it hard to empathise with infertility, a lot of us tend to hide it away, which means that when the grief becomes overwhelming, there is no one to share it with. But if you can find someone to share your story with, do it.

'The four most powerful words you can say are "tell me your story",' says Julia. 'People often come to me thinking they need therapy after pregnancy loss, but quite often I just meet them once or twice. They don't need therapy, they just needed someone to sit there and hear their story through from the beginning to the end. It's through the telling of a story that we integrate experiences into our lives.'

Having someone 'bear witness' to your stories, as she puts it, helps you to acknowledge what has happened to you. 'Some people can feel like they're going a bit mad – they don't feel entitled to their feelings.' Talking about it allows you to 'unpick' your story, she says.

Obviously, if you have a friend or relative you can trust to listen to your story, that's great. If not, there's a British Infertility Counselling Association, and it has a website. We'll put it in the Resources section of this book. Or there's always the 'start a podcast' option. We went for that, and I can testify to the fact that it helped a lot.

Ritual

In 2020 US TV presenter Chrissy Teigen caused uproar by posting photographs of herself giving birth to her stillborn son, Jack. Those who had never experienced the loss of a baby were scandalised: choosing to take photos of such a traumatic event seemed tasteless; choosing to post them online was downright callous. But those who have experienced baby loss understood: every culture has its own version of a mourning ritual, because funerals help those grieving by providing a specific time and place to share memories of the person, which ultimately helps to provide closure, and to mark a new phase of life 'without them'.

When you lose an unborn baby, no one else shares your memories of that person: society never knew they existed – or if it did, it quickly forgets. Finding ways to remind society to acknowledge your baby's existence – however brief, however intangible – can help you to find peace. That could be through photographs of your labour, if that's what you went through, a miscarriage certificate, a funeral (however informal) or a little tree in a garden. It sometimes just helps to remind the world that they were there.

'Chrissy and John [Legend, her husband] have given people permission not to grieve alone,' tweeted writer Ashley C. Ford. 'In the midst of their own deep and enduring pain, they offered a gift to those who know that particular form of heartbreak. Whew! That takes a lot of strength.'

The good news is that the medical community is becoming increasingly good at recognising bereaved parents' need to remember their babies, which is why if you lose a second- or even a first-trimester pregnancy in hospital, it is increasingly common to be provided with a miscarriage certificate, along with a tiny hand- or footprint if your baby was developed enough. Some churches might do memorial services for babies lost in the womb, and 'virtual graveyards' for the unborn exist online.

Even though the baby I lost was no more than an embryo, I choose to remember him (for I am convinced it *was* a 'him') by lighting a candle each year on Pregnancy and Infant Loss Remembrance Day, which is on 15 October each year. Your gesture doesn't have to be grand: it just needs to help you remember.

Conclusion

Loss and grief are, without a doubt, the hardest and most isolating parts of infertility, made all the worse by the fact that society tends to dismiss it. Hopefully, this chapter has given you some idea of what will happen to you physically if you go through a loss, and it will have also helped you to understand what is going on in your head when you are enduring month after month of infertility. Everyone's experiences of these things are different, so don't feel strange if you don't experience any grief at all.

If you're going through it for long enough, counselling is a good option. In the UK, the British Infertility Counselling Association and the UK Council for Psychotherapy can help you find a counsellor or therapist qualified to help those struggling with this type of grief. There are contact details in the back of this book.

13

The Road at the End
of the Road

(Gabby)

Fertility treatment doesn't work for everybody. These are words that none of us want to read, and they're words that we don't want to write. But, sadly, it's the truth. And there can come a time in a couple's fertility journey when they reach something that might feel like a dead end. Perhaps a doctor has advised that further treatment is unlikely to work. Perhaps you'd rather not go through treatment at all. Perhaps one of you is completely exhausted by the process and can't face going through it again. Perhaps it's the money – maybe it's simply the feeling that you've given it your best shot. All these experiences, and many more, are valid and can lead a couple to end their current attempts to start a family.

It might at first feel as though it's the end of your journey to becoming a parent. And that might indeed be true (we'll discuss a way forward in that case later in this chapter). But it doesn't always have to be that way. What can feel like the end of the road can actually be a crossroads of sorts, with options to go a number of different ways. (I'll stop using the road analogy now – this isn't your driving test.)

In this chapter we'll explore four particular options to move forward: donor conception, surrogacy, adoption and living childless. Of course, not everyone who uses these pathways comes to them after failed attempts to conceive; same-sex couples and single parents-to-be will also be considering some of these options. Each of them comes with its own complications and important considerations. We'll learn about each of the processes and we'll also hear from people who have taken these routes.

What you will find in this chapter:

- First steps when it doesn't work.
- Taking care of your emotions with counselling.
- Three makes baby – donor conception.
- Three makes baby – surrogacy.
- The adoption option.
- Childlessness and a different life ahead.

First steps when it doesn't work

Unsuccessful fertility treatment is devastating. Science offers so much hope to those who are trying to create a family, and to find that it hasn't worked for you is nothing short of traumatic. If this is the position you find yourself in, there are a couple of first steps that we recommend taking to ensure that you are in the best position to move forward when the time is right.

Take some time out

For some people, the thought of waiting any longer is unbearable and they don't feel that they need to take any time out. This is completely understandable but there are definitely times in everyone's journey when a bit of downtime, self-care and reflection are really helpful – regardless of what comes next.

You've been through a trauma, and it can be incredibly helpful to allow both your body and your brain to recover, to reflect and to reset. They say 'time is a great healer'. It's very annoying. In fact, giving you a healthy baby would be the best healer of all, thank you very much, but sometimes 'they' are right, and a bit of time out is actually what you (and perhaps your partner) really need. Perhaps it's two weeks, maybe it's two months, maybe it's two years – whatever you decide, it will almost certainly stand you in good stead as you take your next steps.

What should you do in this time? Everyone is different, but talking certainly helps: talk to your partner if you have one, talk to family, talk to friends. Also, don't talk! Take time to be on your own, to process your thoughts and to reconnect with yourself, listen to music, read (non-fertility) books, go for walks – breathe.

You'll probably know when you've had enough of a break, and then you can think about what's next.

Some time on the couch

I'm not talking about your own couch here, although obviously plenty of time on that is also recommended, we're talking about seeking counselling. Nothing can replace the support you need from your partner, friends and family but, often, speaking to someone who specialises in fertility issues, who is removed from your situation, is a really useful thing to do. There might be a counsellor connected to your clinic with whom they can help to organise a meeting for you – or you might need to find one yourself. The British Infertility Counselling Association is a good source to help you find someone local to you who has experience talking about infertility. The HFEA also has a useful page on emotional support, which might be worth a quick look.

When you've decided on your next steps, there might also be required or recommended counselling associated with that. In our opinion, you can never have too much of this. If you've already done a bit of work on getting mentally prepared for what comes next, you'll be in a much better position to make it work.

Three makes baby – donor conception

Donor conception involves the use of donated eggs, sperm (sometimes both) or embryos in order to conceive a child. It is a regularly recommended route for single-sex couples and single people, but also for those who, for whatever reason, aren't producing their own eggs or sperm, or theirs are unlikely to result in pregnancy.

How it works

If this is a route you'd like to pursue, the best place to start is your clinic. As you might imagine, donation isn't a simple process. There's the whole business of finding a donor, there are a lot of health checks and contracts, and, ideally, counselling that need to take place first, and fertility clinics know the drill.

In the UK, it is illegal to pay a donor (other than expenses), which means that donation is purely altruistic. Donors in the UK aren't allowed to remain anonymous, either, which can put people off. It means that waiting lists can be quite long if you're sourcing eggs and sperm in the UK. It's very common for people to look abroad for their eggs and sperm; Spain, for example is a popular place to buy donated eggs, and Denmark is the number-one destination for sperm (there are all sorts of reasons why, but mainly it's a supply-and-demand thing: donors in these countries are paid for their donated genetic materials).

Donated sperm and eggs can be imported from other countries by UK-based clinics, as long as they meet certain conditions. But it's also possible to travel to foreign clinics for treatment using donated eggs or sperm.

If you're having treatment at a licensed fertility clinic in the UK, you can rest assured that your donor will have no legal rights to your kids. You won't ever get your donor's name or address, but when your child is 18, if they want to find the donor, they will be given the necessary details.

Be aware that with home genetic testing (for example, ancestry.com), if your donor-conceived child sends off a mouth swab for DNA analysis and joins the database, contact with the donor or genetic relations can be made in an unregulated way.

Choosing a donor

Whether you're using donated sperm, eggs or embryos, finding the right donor is a huge thing, emotionally and practically. Perhaps you'll want them to look like you, or have certain characteristics, maybe you're interested in their profession, their personality – or simply that they're fit and healthy. For the most part, you can find out some of this information.

For the HFEA to approve donated eggs and sperm they have to meet certain criteria. For women to donate eggs, they must be between 18 and 35 – men must be under 45 to donate sperm – both must not have any family history of genetic disorders or inheritable conditions. In some cases BMI will also be taken into account.

Beyond the basics, you're into personal characteristics. Depending on how you source your eggs or sperm, you will be furnished with an array of info about the donor. Beyond height, weight, hair colour, ethnic background and profession, you might also get interests and their reason for donating, and some clinics ask donors to write a letter to prospective recipients so that they can 'get to know them'. People we've spoken to who have chosen egg and sperm donors have likened the process to online dating, a very strange kind of dating. Don't be surprised if the thing that swings it for you isn't what you expected – what's important is that it feels right.

Sperm donation – the process

If you're buying sperm, once you've found a donor you'd like to use, you can buy a number of vials to use for home insemination, IUI or IVF. You might also decide to reserve that donor's sperm for any future siblings, too.

Some people might also choose to use a known sperm donor – a friend for example – and do a home insemination. The HFEA cautions against this, as the sperm will be untested and you will have to navigate your own complex, almost certainly not legally binding, agreements about rights over the child. Using a known donor, not through the clinic, will automatically make the donor the legal parent.

Egg donation – the process

Once you have chosen your egg donor, it's time to have a discussion about fresh or frozen donation. It depends on the clinic, but some will give you a choice. If you opt for fresh, you and your donor will have to synchronise your cycles before her eggs are collected. You'll probably also take oestrogen to create a lovely womb environment.

If you opt for frozen eggs, the already-collected eggs will be thawed, your partner's or donor's sperm will be used to fertilise the eggs and then an embryo will be transferred. Again, you'll most likely be on oestrogen in the lead-up to transfer.

The donor-egg route: Becky Kearns

Founder of Paths to ParentHub, Becky Kearns has three daughters conceived with donor eggs. Here is her story. When she was diagnosed with early menopause in her late twenties, Becky was told that she might need a donor, but she went through five IVF cycles with her own eggs before coming to the decision. 'Not long after starting IVF we went to a donor conception talk advertised by our clinic to find out more, and it was awful,' she explains. 'There was a mother and grown-up son there who had been conceived through donor sperm, and when he spoke he referred to his dad as 'Clive'. All I could think was that I want my children to call me mum! It terrified me, but in reality I was still in denial and wasn't ready to accept it.'

It wasn't until Becky met a lady who had a little boy through donation that she started to come round to the idea. 'Through meeting her and seeing how she was with her son, I was able to think that actually perhaps it was for me. They were still doing all the things as mother and son that I wanted to do, and there was so much love between them.'

Becky had one more round of IVF with her own eggs, but when it failed she wasn't as devastated as she had been previously. 'The excitement about the possibility with donor eggs was starting to outweigh the grief of not being able to use my eggs,' she explains. Becky and her husband decided to get treatment abroad and flew to Prague for a consultation. 'It suddenly hit me. I started to worry about not being able to see the donor – what would my children look like? And would they have a sixth sense that I wasn't their genetic mum? But we got swept along with it – and it worked first time. I kept a lot of my fears to myself through the pregnancy, but once Mila was born and I had her, that was when it all started to make sense and the decision felt right.'

Becky's advice if you're considering the donor route:

Have counselling first – and not just the mandatory implications session, which can sometimes feel like a tick-box exercise. There can be so much grief connected to the loss of your own eggs or sperm; it's good to work through those issues early on with someone who specialises in donor conception and talk about any fears you have.

Find others who have walked this path If infertility feels lonely, donor conception can feel even lonelier, which is why connection is so important. To build a support network around you find others who truly understand, not only while you're TTC but through pregnancy and parenting, too.

Rehearse your lines Think about how you'll talk to your children about donor conception. I used to talk to Mila about it while she was a baby on the changing mat – she didn't understand, obviously, but it was good practice and I could get upset and it didn't matter. Now we talk about it all the time and we're both really comfortable with it.

Consider the donor's place Remember that the donor will be a presence in your life, but it doesn't have to haunt you. For a while I felt threatened by the idea of our donor, that somehow she could replace me. Now that the girls are here and I'm their mum, I see that even if my girls grow up and want to know about their donor, that doesn't diminish my role as their parent. It's a process of acceptance.

Look into epigenetics and remember the role of nurture I didn't know much about this at the time, but it's really good to understand how this works, because it enables you to focus on what you are contributing rather than what you're not. We can get so hung up on the genetic link that we forget that although the donor might have given you half their genetic blueprint you'll be growing the baby and then teaching them how to be in the world. I see myself in my children through the mannerisms they've picked up from me.

Allow yourself to get excited and visualise your family We all know when you're going through treatment you try not to get too carried away, but if you allow yourself a few moments to imagine what it will be like when you have your baby, including all the little day-to-day, sometimes mundane, things you'll do together, it can really help you to change your mindset about donor conception.

Three makes baby – surrogacy

Surrogacy is an arrangement that sees a woman bear children for someone else. You might be considering surrogacy if you have a tricky womb (terribly technical term, but I prefer it to 'inhospitable', which I find offensive). Perhaps there's a mal-formation, you've had a hysterectomy, you've had recurrent miscarriages, you can't carry a pregnancy due to underlying health conditions, or simply it's a failure for embryos to implant during IVF. Whatever the particulars, sometimes it is recom-mended that embryos from a couple are transferred to another woman's womb.

It is also common for male same-sex couples to start a family this way. A surrogate's eggs (or a donor's eggs) are fertilised with one of the male partner's sperm.

There are two main types of surrogacy:

- Full or host surrogacy, when another woman's eggs are used and there is no genetic link between the carrier and the baby.
- Partial surrogacy, which involves the surrogate's eggs being fertilised by the intended father.

Surrogacy is legal in the UK, but, as we have seen above, you cannot pay a surrogate, unless it is their expenses. For this reason, surrogacy in the UK is an altruistic act and so it often happens between people who already know each other. That's not to say if friends and family aren't an option, you can't find someone. Your clinic is not allowed to find a surrogate for you. But there are organisations that can help. These are good places to start:

- Surrogacy UK
- Brilliant Beginnings
- My Surrogacy Journey
- Childlessness Overcome Through Surrogacy (COTS)

The legality

The legality surrounding surrogacy in the UK is a bit tricky (to say the least). Unfortunately, surrogacy agreements can be put in place, but they are not enforceable by UK law. Also, the surrogate is the legal mother of the child until you get a parental order from the court, even if the surrogate is not genetically related to the child. This sounds very scary, but it's not the end of the world, it just means a bit of extra paperwork at the start. Once the parental order is in place, the surrogate will not have any rights with regards to the child.

There is also the possibility of nominating a legal second parent at birth: if the surrogate is married or in a civil partnership, her partner will automatically be the legal second parent (until you've got your parental order in place). But if she is single, the man providing the sperm will automatically be the legal second parent at birth. The surrogate is able to nominate a legal second parent at birth. You need to get this in place before the embryo is transferred.

It is a bit of a legal minefield, so we definitely recommend seeking legal counsel, but you can certainly start with your clinic, which should be able to explain the basics.

The surrogacy route: Ginanne Brownell

Journalist and author of *How I Became Your Mother: My Global Surrogacy Journey*, Ginanne Brownell has twins – a son and a daughter – born through an egg donor and surrogate. Here is her story: Ginanne was at Wimbledon the day before her last egg collection when her doctor called to say that if it didn't work, she should consider stopping IVF. 'There I was, under the stairs silently sobbing while everyone was cheering and shouting as Rafael Nadal scored an amazing point. Sure enough, we did the transfer, and it didn't work.'

Ginanne and her husband knew that they wanted kids, and because they still had frozen embryos left over, they started looking into surrogacy. 'A real turning point for me was when I was talking to two middle-class, gay friends of mine who live in Israel and were going through the process of surrogacy,' she says. 'Until that point, it had seemed to me like something only rich and famous people did. But here were my friends doing it, and they explained the process to me and gradually I became more comfortable.'

They decided to find a surrogate in Ginanne's native US. 'Firstly, I'm American and secondly, I felt more comfortable with the ethics of surrogacy in the US. It's very different in countries across the globe; there are more developed countries with pretty high standards, but there are some places where we weren't sure how the surrogate was going to be treated.'

They found an agency called Circle – the largest surrogacy agency in the US and also a family formation law firm. 'I quite liked that idea. It was important to me that the surrogates were empowered.' The couple ended up on a blind date with a surrogate called Julie. She had a master's degree, ran a not-for-profit company and lived in Illinois – very close to Ginanne's mum.

Sadly, the embryos they already had didn't work. 'We transferred two blasts, which didn't take and then a third, which got her pregnant but she miscarried at eight weeks. Our contract said we could try to use our surrogate only three times, so we thought, right, what now?!'

They went back to their agency, which found an egg donor for them. Eventually they transferred embryos and the first time they actually met Julie face to face she was 12 weeks pregnant with their twins. 'We all went to a Chicago Cubs game and she waddled down the stairs to our seats, and I was like "Oh my God, she's carrying our babies!"'

When the babies were eventually born via C-section, Ginanne recalls a very surreal moment in the hospital. 'Only one person was allowed in the room, and she wanted her husband because it was obviously a big surgery,' explains Ginanne. 'So while my kids were being born, I was in a cafeteria eating a ham sandwich. When I started the sandwich I was just me, when I finished it, I was a mum.'

Ginanne's advice if you're considering surrogacy:

Do your due diligence 'Different countries have different rules, and it's important to understand how you and your surrogate will be impacted by them. Here's a little simple checklist of things to look out for:

1   Your rights as the mother and the legal framework supporting that.
2   The treatment of the surrogate and their understanding of the undertaking.

3　The strength of the contracts in place to protect you both.

4　The legality of surrogacy where you live and where you choose to do it.

Understand that you will have complex emotions towards your surrogate 'It's a very strange situation to be in. Another woman is walking about growing your child. But our surrogate said something wonderful: she said she felt that she considered it to be like intense babysitting and was merely minding my babies for nine months.'

Know that your feelings might change 'At one point, my egg donor reached out to our agency asking to see photos of the babies, and my mama-bear instinct said "No way!" Since writing my book, I have come to realise the importance of that link to their donor. I wrote to her to say my mind had changed and I would like to keep the line of communication open.'

Your labour is just as valid – 'sure, you're not carrying the baby/babies, and you won't give birth to them, but you have been through labour – just a different kind. The struggle to get to this point is *your* labour. My labour wasn't physical, but it was complex and emotional.'

The adoption option

We have no doubt that you're sick to the back teeth of people saying, 'Why don't you just adopt?' It feels like a frustration that anyone going through infertility must endure – but that's not to say that adoption isn't a valid option. The reason that phrase is so hard to stomach is (a) you must first get your head around not having a biological child; and (b) there's no 'just' about it: it's very bloody complex.

If you think adoption might be for you, it's a good idea to attend some information events – hear a bit more about the process and the kinds of things you need to consider before heading into it. If you've done this and you'd like to proceed, it's time to choose an agency. There are all sorts of options in the UK, from local councils to charities such as Barnardo's. Speak to as many as possible and get a feel for who you'd like to work with. These people will be digging into your life, so it's a good idea that you don't hate them.

Once you've settled on which route you want to go down, you'll enter into the evaluation process (the aforementioned digging) where the agency will conduct a lot of background checks and you'll probably make lots of cakes for visiting social workers. They will eventually submit your file to an adoption panel which will decide whether you're suitable to adopt.

Hopefully, you'll get accepted and the agency will start the process of matching you with a child. You'll probably go through a lot of profiles before you find a good match for you, and if all is well on both sides, you'll start introductions. The child spends increasing amounts of time with you until, eventually, they stay for good.

Not a Fictional Mum (NFM)

Adoption blogger NFM (who doesn't share her name) has one son through adoption, is currently in the process of adopting another child, and launched her blog and online shop to help adoptive parents feel less alone and less 'fictional'. Here is her story. NFM is determined to share her story because she wants to change the narrative around adoption as a last resort. She and her husband tried fertility treatment before adopting their son, 'because that's the next path a lot of people take. When IVF didn't work, we started to think: *Why did we want this in the first place?* We want to grow our family. We want to love and nurture a child, so can we not do this another way? So we explored adoption.'

The first steps to meeting their son

The couple started by going to information evenings, something NFM says is necessary because although this route to parenthood is beautiful, it is challenging. 'There are other families involved that aren't going to disappear – they will rightfully be part of a child's life, in their history, forever. So understanding all of this first is essential.' They decided to go with Barnardo's because of the support the charity offers. They also decided that rather than try to adopt a very young baby, known as early permanence, they would go for a slightly older child.

'One thing that becomes very apparent in the world of adoption is that you get very limited information about a child the younger they are,' she explains. 'Of course, there is uncertainty with any adoption, but with very little health and development information available for tiny babies, you have to ask yourself whether you could handle that level of uncertainty? And we couldn't. Our little boy was 21 months when he came to us, so if we hadn't made that decision not to opt for early permanence we wouldn't have found him.'

Finding him

Once they were approved to adopt, they entered the family-finding process. NFM describes this as one of the hardest parts. 'It feels a little inhuman,' she says. 'There is basically a website where you go, and there are lots of children's profiles on there and you spend your evenings scrolling through. When you think you've found a match that you feel could work for you, you let the charity know.'

They were the last couple in their group to find a match, but when they saw their son's profile they knew. 'My husband shouted, "I've found him!" He had this beautiful curly hair, lovely eyes and it was all about his personality – he loved dancing, having his photo taken, loved cheese! And was cheeky. I just thought: *We're meant to be!*'

Bringing him home

Once they expressed interest, the couple had more visits from social workers – 'house is clean, but not too clean – you don't want to appear neurotic'. Eventually they heard that of all the couples who had expressed interest in their little boy, they had been chosen. They began a period of introductions, until eventually he came to live in his 'forever home'.

'You might imagine the day the foster carers go is a happy day,' says NFM, 'that you close the door and that's it – but he was absolutely heartbroken and grieved for weeks and weeks after that. All we could do was show him as much love as possible. You're asking a child to start loving someone all over again. It's not a fairy tale. But it is worth it.'

NFM says it took a while to fall completely in love – after

all he was a stranger. But eventually they did, and there was no turning back. 'It's bizarre with adoption because I think there is a higher plane of love. If you have experienced pain – and if you've been through infertility, you know pain – and there is a little child that is experiencing pain, there's an empathy and connection that you have with each other.

'Now I think: *God! Imagine if fertility treatment had worked! We might never have met this amazing human and I might not be a mum to this little boy.*'

Things to keep in mind

The birth family will always be a part of your child's history Your child will come to you with his or her history and it's important to embrace it, says NFM. 'When you look at the adoption symbol it is a triangle – representing the birth family, the adoptive family and the child. We are all part of this child's life in some capacity. We don't have too much contact with the birth family; we write a letter once a year, but we don't share photos or anything else. But we don't shy away from them as part of my son's life.'

It is challenging but rewarding People are very nervous about it and no one should be talked into adoption – it is massive and it's challenging, says NFM. 'But there is nothing more rewarding than when a child looks at you and tells you that they love you and they really believe that you love them back. They have chosen to love you – it's not something they have to do, it's not biological, and they've been on a journey as you have.'

Childlessness and a different life ahead

Childlessness is a very negative word. It feels very harsh, somehow. But, actually, deciding to remain childless after a period of infertility and all the trauma and emotional exhaustion it brings with it can become an empowering resolution to a very difficult part of your life. Some like to use the phrase 'child-free' instead of childless – it strikes a more positive tone. But others feel that this is a phrase better suited to those who have never wanted kids, because somehow child-free erases their struggle. Everyone is different.

In this section, we'll use 'childless not by choice', sometimes seen as the acronym CNBC on Internet forums.

There are many reasons a couple might decide to live childless not by choice. It has a lot to do with reaching a predetermined 'end point'. Perhaps you said you'd stop trying when you reached a certain age, a certain number of treatments, when the money or your emotional energy runs out. All these are valid and no one is going to rush you in coming to this point. Rather than entering a system or process with a series of defined milestones, like some of the other options we've discussed, childless not by choice is a decision that requires you to do some work on yourself. You need to give yourself time to grieve before you can start to come to terms with and embrace a different life than you had imagined.

Getting help: Gateway Women

Gateway Women started as a blog by Jody Day, because she couldn't find any support about her decision to be CNBC. When other women started to get in touch, it grew from there. It is a support network for women grieving the loss of motherhood. Gateway Women is for those who are permanently involuntarily childless – for any reason at all. It is an online community, with a platform to share feelings and ask questions: 'If you're having a bad day and just want to vent, we're all there for each other with words of encouragement,' says one of Gateway Women's Reignite Weekend facilitators, Yvonne John.

There is also a range of resources. The Reignite Weekend, for example, is hosted over two days. Over the course of the weekend the team works through past and present grief, before moving on to imagine moving forward and 'reigniting your spark of joy'. 'When you're really deep in the grief, you can get stuck,' says Yvonne. 'It's very sad and heavy. Often friends and family can't really help because they just want to fix you but they don't understand how. We take a close look at where you are, why you're stuck there and create a space to let it out (not let it go).'

As well as working for Gateway Women, Yvonne John is author of *Dreaming of a Life Unlived*. This is her story: Yvonne got married at 39 and started trying for a baby because she didn't want to hit the menopause without having a go. 'I was pretty ambivalent about being a mum,' she explains. 'Part of me felt it was probably too late anyway – I don't remember having much hope. But after three years of trying something had changed.'

The process of TTC started to take its toll on Yvonne. She decided to go for investigations, but the doctors weren't particularly helpful. 'First they said, "Why didn't you try sooner?" Helpful. Then they said, "Well we can't see anything wrong with you, you have unexplained infertility, just keep trying." I remember thinking in my heart: *It just isn't going to happen.* And instantly, I was very sad.'

Yvonne was struggling to come to terms with the situation,

avoiding mothers and pregnant women (we all know the drill), when her friend directed her to Gateway Women. She did her first workshop in December 2014. 'My first thought was that there was no way I could share my story with the women there,' she says. 'I had terminations in my early twenties and I thought that they would never accept me. But all I got was love and acceptance. I ended up doing a 12-month mentorship programme. It was amazing and helped me to find my normality again – self-acceptance and forgiving my younger self was a huge thing.' Recognising her feelings as grief was a huge part of the process. 'I also felt I didn't deserve to grieve because of my past. But to be around women who accepted it, understood it and named it "grief" was huge.'

Seven years on, Yvonne still feels it but not as deeply as before. She has coping mechanisms and strategies, and knows what her triggers are. 'I have learned how to make choices that best suit me,' she explains. 'If I am invited to a family event, I know I can say no, or I can go and give myself permission to leave if I need to. The process has given me the strength to own my story. It doesn't take the wind out of my lungs when someone asks if I have children any more. I can answer in any way I feel – or not at all.'

Conclusion

Not many people start their fertility journey hoping to end up using one of these further options. But for the most part, those who do and find success in a way they hadn't at first imagined wouldn't change things for the world. Whether people have adopted children, or conceived through a donor or a surrogate, all routes to parenthood look different, and we should celebrate and embrace that.

Of course, there are also couples who don't end up having children – we hope that this chapter has helped to shed light on what that life might look like and how you can come to terms with a different path than the one you hoped for.

The End of this Jourrrney

The first time we sat down together with a microphone and started telling our stories it was like a switch was flicked. Suddenly the baggage we were carrying around got a little lighter, the sadness that always seemed to be there drifted off. And in its place were belly laughs. Big deep belly laughs. We laughed at the inevitable embarrassment of internal scans, we laughed at the wave of pregnancy announcements hitting us like smacks in the face, we laughed at sperm samples going missing, we laughed at the number of people who had seen our lady parts that week.

There are many things that we hope you have taken from this book. But one of the biggest is the power of these belly laughs. They are important to us. For some, it might feel somehow crass to make jokes about something as serious as infertility. Perhaps we aren't treating the situation with the kid gloves it requires. But we believe that laughing is actually the best weapon anyone has against infertility.

When you're on this jourrrney, it can feel like you're completely out of control. Like all these horrible, unfortunate and damn unfair things keep happening to you. They knock you down, time and time again, blow after blow. But if you can take these things and own them – use them as hilarious anecdotes in the pub, write a comedic entry in your private diary at the end of the day or give your partner a giggle on the couch, you start to take on control of them. They aren't pushing you around any more – you're pushing them. And we can say from experience that it makes everything feel a bit better.

We also hope that this book has given you the power of knowledge. Infertility can be a steep learning curve – from how your body works to how science can help it – it's bamboozling at times, but it doesn't have to be. We hope you can use this book as a guide, something you pick up at different stages of your jourrrney that gives you a head start on what to expect and the questions you might want to ask.

Last but, by all of the means possible, not least, we hope that this book has made you feel less alone. Because, above all else, the thing that makes infertility so hard is the fact that it seems you're the only person in the world going through it.

Instagram, Facebook, your friends' WhatsApp group, your mum's updates from home – these interactions with the people we know are littered with pregnancy announcements, new baby pictures, first day at school shots. But you can't join in. No matter how hard you try. And it hurts. No wonder it can feel like you're going mad.

Let us say this: *you're not alone*. And you're not crazy. The problem, as we've said before, is that no one talks about infertility. We've been on a mission from day one to shout about it from the rooftops. Because, as we see it, the more we talk the less shame there will be around something you have no control over. Sure, the infertility club is a club that no one wants to be a part of – but lots of people are, so let's talk.

You don't have to start a podcast, you don't have to write a book, but talking about it, even with just one other person, will make it so much easier. So remember, the first rule of infertility club? You *do* talk about infertility club. Second rule of infertility club? You *do* talk about infertility club. Third rule of infertility club? Err, tell all your friends to buy our book. Winky emoji.

And so, here ends our jourrrney together (for now).

Glossary

3dpo (for example): three days past ovulation; slang used on Internet forums.

3dp5dt (for example): three days past five-day transfer. Refers to the amount of time that has passed since an embryo transfer, and how 'old' that embryo is. Again, slang used on Internet forums.

AF: Aunt Flo – another term for a period.

Agonist/antagonist: see 'protocol'.

AMH: anti-Müllerian hormone.

Asthenozoospermia: sperm with bad motility (see below).

Azoospermia: the medical condition describing a man who has zero sperm in his ejaculate.

Baseline scan: an ultrasound scan, usually internal, which is performed at the beginning of an IVF or transfer cycle to check your ovaries and uterus.

BFN: big fat negative (aka negative pregnancy test).

BFP: big fat positive (aka positive pregnancy test).

Blastocyst: the stage an embryo reaches about five days after fertilisation, when there are too many cells to count.

Body temperature, basal/core: some women check their temperature every day to determine where they are in their cycle. Basal temperature is your temperature when you are fully at rest; core temperature is measured by inserting a thermometer into your vagina or rectum.

CCG: Clinical Commissioning Group: your local NHS funding body.

Cervical mucus/secretions: the 'discharge' secreted by your cervix during the first part of your menstrual cycle.

Cervix: the 'neck' of the uterus, made up of muscle, which connects the vagina and the uterus.

Chemical pregnancy: the name given to a miscarriage in the very earliest stages of pregnancy, usually shortly after implantation.

Chromosomes: structures inside cells, made up of protein and DNA, which tell the cells how to grow. Humans have 23 'pairs', or karyotypes, of chromosomes.

Clomid, clomifene citrate: a drug designed to stimulate ovulation in women with PCOS.

Corpus luteum: the body left behind in the ovary after ovulation, which secretes progesterone.

Crusty jazz mags: old porn magazines with suspected sperm stains, usually found in clinics.

Cycle: the menstrual cycle describes a woman's 'monthly' cycle between ovulation and menstruation. An IVF cycle is usually a round of drugs, egg collection, then transfer of any resulting embryos, although this definition tends to differ, depending on your clinic.

Date with Wanda: (see 'internal ultrasound scan').

Dildocam: (see 'internal ultrasound scan').

DNA fragmentation: abnormal genetic material in sperm, which can lead to a higher chance of pregnancy loss or failed implantation.

Ectopic pregnancy: this occurs when the fertilised egg implants somewhere other than the uterus, most often in the Fallopian tubes. Ectopic pregnancy always results in pregnancy loss, and can be life-threatening.

Egg retrieval/collection: the process of retrieving eggs from the ovaries during an IVF cycle using a catheter, which is inserted up through the vagina, then through the uterine wall. This is usually performed under 'heavy sedation'.

Embryo: the very earliest stages of a baby. It stays an embryo until the eleventh week of pregnancy, when it becomes a foetus.

Embryo grading: the process of figuring out the quality of an embryo, based on the shape and evenness of its cells (see Chapter 8).

Embryologist: a scientist working on the lab side of IVF. Their job includes collecting eggs, preparing sperm samples, injecting sperm into eggs, culturing embryos and performing embryo biopsies.

Endometriosis: a condition where tissue similar to the womb lining grows in places outside the uterus, causing excruciating pain. It can cause fertility complications.

Endometrium/endometrial lining/womb lining: the lining of the uterus, which grows once a month and is then shed during the period.

Fallopian tubes: the tiny tubes that carry the egg from the ovaries to the uterus.

Fertile window: the time around ovulation when you should be able to conceive. Although the egg survives for 12–14 hours after ovulation, the fertile window is longer because sperm can survive in the uterus for up to five days.

Fertility awareness: the practice of monitoring various signals in your body to work out when you are most likely to conceive.

Fibroids: growths that develop in or around the uterus, which can lead to fertility complications.

FMU: first-morning urine. First thing in the morning is usually when your urine is at its most concentrated, meaning that pregnancy or ovulation tests will be most accurate.

Follicle: the tiny sacs inside ovaries that have the potential to release an egg during ovulation. After ovulation, the collapsed follicle becomes a corpus luteum, which secretes progesterone.

Frozen embryo transfer (FET): the procedure during which a thawed-out frozen embryo is placed into the uterus by a doctor.

FSH: follicle stimulating hormone. FSH is a pituitary hormone that stimulates the growth of follicles in the ovary before ovulation (see Chapter 1).

Hatching embryo: at the early stages of development, an embryo is made up of a ball of cells, known as an inner cell mass (ICM), surrounded by a 'shell' called the zona pellucida. After five or six days, the ICM should begin to break out of the zona pellucida (see Chapter 8).

HFEA: Human Fertilisation and Embryology Authority, the UK regulator overseeing fertility treatment and clinics.

HSG, HyCoSy: a hysterosalpingogram (HSG) or hysterosalpingo contrast sonography (HyCoSy) is a test in which dye is flushed through the Fallopian tubes to check their 'patency', or how open they are. The only difference is how the dye is watched: in an HSG, it's done under an X-ray, whereas in a HyCoSy it's done via an ultrasound.

Hughes syndrome, antiphospholipid syndrome, sticky blood: a blood-clotting disorder that has been linked to recurrent pregnancy loss, late pregnancy loss, stillbirth and a range of other pregnancy complications.

Human chorionic gonadotropin (hCG): although hCG is present in the body in small amounts most of the time, it is known as the 'pregnancy hormone' because it is produced in larger quantities by the embryo once it has implanted in the uterus. This is the hormone pregnancy tests look for.

Hysteroscopy: a procedure where a tiny camera is inserted into the uterus to assess it and check for abnormalities.

ICSI: intra-cytoplasmic sperm injection. The process of selecting the best sperm and injecting it into an egg to fertilise it. This is usually used to treat male-factor infertility.

Immunotherapy: a relatively new field of medicine treating high levels of natural killer cells (NK cells, see below) in the endometrium. Evidence for the efficacy of this is still relatively weak.

Implantation: the moment an embryo attaches itself to the wall of the uterus.

Implantation bleeding: very, very light spotting that is thought to occur when an embryo implants.

Inner cell mass, ICM: (see 'hatching').

Internal ultrasound scan: also known as a 'date with Wanda' or 'dildocam'. This is when a nurse uses a dildo-shaped ultrasound scanner to get a better look at the uterus, ovaries and Fallopian tubes. This shouldn't be an uncomfortable procedure.

IUI: intra-uterine insemination. When a doctor inserts sperm directly into the uterus, bypassing the cervix. This is much cheaper than IVF, but it has lower success rates.

IVF: in-vitro fertilisation. The blanket term given to the process of artificially removing one or more eggs from the ovaries, fertilising them artificially, then inserting the resulting embryo into the uterus.

Laparoscopy: a procedure where a surgeon looks at the inside of the abdomen using a tiny camera, which is inserted through a tiny incision in the skin. In fertility, it's often used to assess – and sometimes clip or remove – the Fallopian tubes, or remove cysts from the ovaries.

Letrozole: a drug designed to treat breast cancer in post-menopausal women, it is also prescribed to help PCOS sufferers to ovulate.

Line eyes: that fuzzy vision you get when you're staring at a pregnancy test too hard. Is that the ghost of a second line, or is it a shadow?

Luteal phase: the part of the menstrual cycle after ovulation, but before the period.

Luteal support: the term given to the drugs provided to help the body create the right conditions for pregnancy after an embryo is transferred. This usually takes the form of progesterone.

Luteinising hormone (LH): a hormone produced by the pituitary gland, which surges just before ovulation, causing the ovary to release a mature egg.

Metformin: a drug designed for type-2 diabetes patients to lower insulin resistance, which is often prescribed to PCOS sufferers to help regulate their cycles.

MFI: male-factor infertility.

Morphology: the shape and regularity of something; for example, an embryo or a sperm.

Motility: the ability (of sperm) to move normally.

Natural killer (NK) cells: a type of white blood cell produced by the bone marrow which are present in the uterine lining. It's thought that abnormal NK cells might have an effect on embryo implantation, although the evidence for this is still weak (see 'Immunotherapy').

NICE: National Institute for Health and Care Excellence. The UK body producing evidence-based guidelines for those operating in medical fields, including fertility.

Oestrogen: the hormone that controls the development and release of the egg each cycle and causes the uterine lining to thicken during the first half of the cycle.

OHSS: ovarian hyperstimulation syndrome. Iatrogenic disease caused by the over-stimulation of the ovaries using IVF drugs. In very rare cases, it results in the death of a patient.

OPK: ovulation predictor kit. A strip of plastic that works in a similar way to a pregnancy test, in that you pee on it, but it measures luteinising hormone so that you can time sex to coincide with the pre-ovulation surge. It costs a lot in shops but simple versions are much cheaper on Amazon.

OTD: official test day. The day your clinic (or your cycle) decrees that you must either take a home pregnancy test or a blood test to determine whether TTC or an IVF cycle has worked. You *will* be up at 5am.

Ovaries: female reproductive organs that produce eggs and secrete oestrogen and progesterone.

Ovulation: the release of a mature egg by an ovary, which should take place in the middle of the menstrual cycle.

PCOS: polycystic ovary syndrome. The name given to a condition affecting one in ten women that prevents ovulation from taking place regularly. Signs include irregular periods, hirsutism and 'cysts' on the ovaries, which can be seen on an ultrasound. The condition can cause complications with fertility. You can also have polycystic ovaries without the 'syndrome' (known as PCO) (see Chapter 6).

PGT-A (previously PGS): pre-implantation genetic testing for aneuploidy. Procedure where a biopsy is taken from a blastocyst, then checked for chromosomal abnormalities.

PGT-M (previously PGD): pre-implantation genetic testing for monogenic/single gene defects. A procedure where a biopsy is taken from a blastocyst, then checked for single gene disorders such as cystic fibrosis, sickle cell disease, beta thalassemia or the BRCA 1 or 2 genes. This is used for parents who are at a high risk of passing on a disorder they are known to carry.

PGT-SR (previously PGD): pre-implantation genetic testing for chromosomal structural rearrangements. A procedure where a biopsy is taken from a blastocyst, then checked for normal size or arrangement of chromosomes. This is used for parents with chromosome rearrangements such as a balanced translocation, who are at risk of producing children with the incorrect amount of genetic material.

Placenta: an organ that develops alongside a baby in the uterus which provides oxygen and nutrients to the baby.

POAS: pee on a stick – to take a pregnancy test.

Progesterone: hormone produced by the corpus luteum (see above) after ovulation, which thickens the uterine lining and eventually supports a pregnancy.

Pregnancy loss, miscarriage: the loss of a baby during pregnancy. After 12 weeks of pregnancy it is known as a late miscarriage; after 24 weeks it is a stillbirth.

Protocol: the drugs regime used during an IVF cycle. These are usually a long 'agonist' protocol, during which your ovaries are 'down-regulated' over several weeks, or a short 'antagonist' protocol, during which your ovaries are shut down more quickly (see Chapter 8).

PUPO: pregnant until proven otherwise – a woman's condition following embryo transfer.

TTC: trying to conceive.

Speculum: device used to hold open the vagina during a variety of unpleasant and undignified procedures.

Spotting: small amounts of vaginal bleeding outside your period. Warning: can lead to excess crying.

Stillbirth: the death of a baby in utero after 24 weeks of pregnancy.

Stims: drugs used to stimulate your ovaries during an IVF cycle – usually either pure FSH or a mixture of FSH and LH (see Chapter 8).

Subfertility: a delay in conceiving – but the possibility of a natural conception is still there.

Trigger shot: the final injection during an IVF stim cycle, which is taken 36 hours before egg retrieval and tells your ovaries to release their eggs. Usually this is made up of hCG, although it can also be an agonist drug.

Unexplained infertility: the most frustrating diagnosis where clinicians recognise you aren't conceiving but can't figure out why.

Uterine abnormalities (bicornuate, unicornuate, septate, subseptate, arcuate): a uterus that is unusually shaped. See Chapter 4 for descriptions.

Vagina: the canal connecting the vulva with the cervix.

Vulva: the external part of the female genitals.

Resources

TTC basics

Fertility Network UK: https://fertilitynetworkuk.org/. For UK
readers, their helpline number is 01424 732361
NICE guidelines on infertility: https://www.nice.org.uk/
guidance/cg156
If you're interested in the Fertility Awareness Method, check
out Lisa Hendrickson-Jack's book, *The Fifth Vital Sign*.
Her podcast is called Fertility Friday and is available on
all good platforms and at https://fertilityfriday.com/
Joyce Harper's book, *Your Fertile Years*, is a great read
whether you're TTC or not.

Mental health and support

Alice Rose's mindset reset: https://www.thisisalicerose.com/
reclaim
British Infertility Counselling Association: https://www.bica.net/

IVF Babble: https://www.ivfbabble.com/

Kezia Okafor: https://keziaokafor.com/

Meditation support: https://www.headspace.com/ and
        https://www.mindfulivf.com/

Shirlee Kay, the sex therapist who specialises in infertility:
        https://www.shirleekay.co.uk/

UK Council for Psychotherapy: https://www.psychotherapy.
        org.uk/

Grief and pregnancy loss

ARC, a charity supporting parents through antenatal screening,
        and any terminations that might result from that: https://
        arc-uk.org/

Julia Bueno's wonderful book on pregnancy and baby loss,
        The Brink of Being, is available from all good bookshops.
        Her website is http://www.juliabueno.co.uk/

Miscarriage Association:
        https://www.miscarriageassociation.org.uk/

PETALS (Pregnancy Expectations Trauma and Loss Society):
        https://petalscharity.org/

Tommy's: https://www.tommys.org/

Preparing for IVF

Access Fertility: https://www.accessfertility.com/

HFEA: https://www.hfea.gov.uk/ (includes clinic reviews and
        the traffic light system)

Fertility nurse and consultant Kate Davies:
        https://yourfertilityjourney.com/

Nutritionist Melanie Brown:
    https://melaniebrownnutrition.com/
Your IVF Abroad: https://www.yourivfabroad.co.uk/
People are always asking us for the name of our acupuncturist.
    She's called Lui Yeung, and you can find her at
    https://www.luiacupuncture.com/
There are loads of videos on self-injecting at
    https://ivflondon.co.uk/self-injecting/

The road at the end of the road

Adoption: https://www.adoptionuk.org/ and
    https://notafictionalmum.com/
Childlessness: https://gateway-women.com/
Donor conception: Paths to ParentHub – https://members.
    definingmum.com/ and Donor conception network –
    https://www.dcnetwork.org/
Surrogacy: https://www.brilliantbeginnings.co.uk/ and
    https://surrogacyuk.org/

Pregnancy after infertility

Cat Strawbridge's Finally Pregnant podcast can be found on
    all podcast platforms
Pregnancy After Loss Support:
    https://pregnancyafterlosssupport.org/
Zoe Clark-Coats' book *Pregnancy after Loss* is available from
    all good bookshops.

Additional resources

Fertility Matters At Work: http://instagram.com/
    fertilitymattersatwork
Fertility Network UK: https://fertilitynetworkuk.org/
    trying-to-conceive/fertility-at-work/

Index

Acknowledgements

Thank you, first and foremost, to Maria Whelan of Inkwell for spotting two whiny podcasters and believing they could write a book, and to Juliet Pickering of Blake Friedmann, who has been so gentle and tender throughout the process.

Big thanks also go to Zoe Bohm, Jillian Stewart and the rest of the Piatkus team, who took a leap of faith when they decided to publish this book, and are among the most generous editors either of us have worked with.

A million thank-yous to all of the contributors in this book, whose time, thoughts and feelings have made the book richer – we're sure your stories and advice will help many, and we're delighted to be able to share them.

Thank you to Professor Tim and Jonathan Ramsay for reading the WHOLE book and not only helping us to make it better but also telling us how much you liked it. *Blushing faces*. And to Julia Bueno, whose help with the chapter on pregnancy loss was invaluable.

Big love to Mr Gabby and Mr Emma (AKA Mr BFN Art Director and Mr BFN photographer), whose enthusiasm and support has never once wavered, except occasionally in the direction of *over*-enthusiasm, which is the correct direction. When we've been stressed and we've doubted we could do it, you've furnished us with confidence and white wine.

To The Foxes, Liz and Nick, and BFN Sophie for joining the gang, bearing your souls and being our constant cheerleaders.

To Sophie, Emma's BFF, who didn't bat an eyelid about sharing our worst-ever argument because it might help someone. To Jane and her most brilliant and important fiancé Dan, for letting Gabby share the time they were newly pregnant and Gabby embarrassed herself.

Thank you to our mums and dads, brothers and sisters, who mopped up tears, gave hugs and provided chocolate throughout both our 'journeyyyys', and to our friends, some of whom endured us disappearing from their lives altogether while we tried to get our heads around what was happening to us.

And, of course, Noah and Otis, who gave us our happy endings. Your contributions to the initial publishers meeting, at approximately six months and six weeks old respectively, were vital. We hope you'll forgive us for talking about every moment of your conception and mentioning the phrase dildocam too many times for a parent.

The final, most important thanks go to our listeners, subscribers and you – our readers. You have fiercely supported us since that very first episode, back in 2018, when we declared in wobbly voices that we wanted to change the way infertility is talked about. We haven't always got it right, but you've forgiven us and you've grown with us. We are grateful to every single one of you. Thank you, thank you, thank you.